Women and Girls with Autism Spectrum Disorder

by the same author

The Adolescent and Adult Neuro-diversity Handbook
Asperger Syndrome, ADHD, Dyslexia, Dyspraxia and Related Conditions
Sarah Hendrickx with Claire Salter
ISBN 978 1 84310 980 8
eISBN 978 0 85700 220 4

Love, Sex and Long-term Relationships
What People with Asperger Syndrome Really Really Want
Sarah Hendrickx
Foreword by Stephen M. Shore
ISBN 978 1 84310 605 0
eISBN 978 1 84642 764 0

Asperger Syndrome and Employment
What People with Asperger Syndrome Really Really Want
Sarah Hendrickx
ISBN 978 1 84310 677 7
eISBN 978 1 84642 879 1

Asperger Syndrome – A Love Story
Sarah Hendrickx and Keith Newton
Foreword by Tony Attwood
ISBN 978 1 84310 540 4
eISBN 978 1 84642 662 9

Asperger Syndrome and Alcohol
Drinking to Cope?
Matthew Tinsley and Sarah Hendrickx
Foreword by Temple Grandin
ISBN 978 1 84310 609 8
eISBN 978 1 84642 814 2

of related interest

Aspergirls
Empowering Females with Asperger Syndrome
Rudy Simone
Foreword by Liane Holliday Willey
ISBN 978 1 84905 826 1
eISBN 978 0 85700 289 1

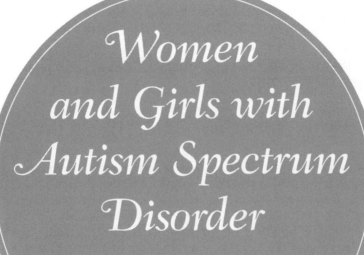

Women and Girls with Autism Spectrum Disorder

UNDERSTANDING LIFE EXPERIENCES FROM EARLY CHILDHOOD TO OLD AGE

Sarah Hendrickx

Foreword by Dr Judith Gould

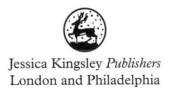

Jessica Kingsley *Publishers*
London and Philadelphia

First published in 2015
by Jessica Kingsley Publishers
73 Collier Street
London N1 9BE, UK
and
400 Market Street, Suite 400
Philadelphia, PA 19106, USA

www.jkp.com

Library of Congress Cataloging in Publication Data
A CIP catalog record for this book is available from the Library of Congress

British Library Cataloguing in Publication Data
A CIP catalogue record for this book is available from the British Library

ISBN 978 1 84905 547 5
eISBN 978 0 85700 982 1

Printed and bound in Great Britain

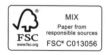

MIX
Paper from
responsible sources
FSC
www.fsc.org   FSC® C013056

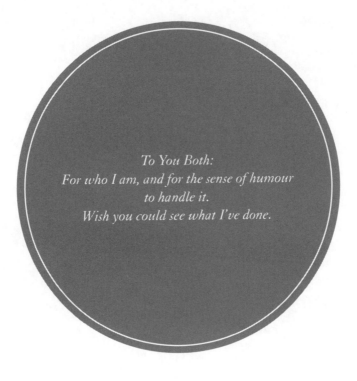

To You Both:
For who I am, and for the sense of humour
to handle it.
Wish you could see what I've done.

Contents

Foreword

DR JUDITH GOULD

Historically there has been an assumption that autism is predominantly a male condition.

The female pattern of behaviour in classic autism was clear in those who were intellectually disabled but the girls and women who were more verbal and intellectually able were missed. It is only in recent years that we have begun to recognise the female presentation of behaviours in the autism spectrum and there are now many books written on this subject, usually by women on the spectrum. This book adds to our knowledge by providing an insightful, sensitive analysis of the pattern of behaviours in females from childhood through to old age.

The author poses the question 'Why did I write the book?' She, like so many other women, has experienced the disbelief of professionals who have a narrow, stereotyped view of the male pattern of behaviour. She questions that autism is diagnosed on behaviour patterns when these are often different in women. The way forward is not that we need a new set of diagnostic criteria but a better understanding of how the behaviours are manifested in women. A book such as this is a useful resource in understanding the complexities of the female presentation of the condition.

This book combines existing research and knowledge on the subject, backed up with the personal experiences of women with autism and the families of girls with autism. Throughout, the examples given provide invaluable insights into the way the women and girls think.

The review of research sets the scene and the conclusion is that autism is more diverse than originally thought, with new ideas being put forward every day. In fact, it's a case of 'the more we know, the less we know', particularly in how gender affects individuals with autism. Overall, there is little research differentiating the male/female profile. We are yet to establish an accurate estimate of the prevalence of the male:female ratio. If women are not being diagnosed then we cannot reliably say what the ratio is likely to be. Getting a diagnosis is covered in this book, which clearly sets out the difficulties experienced by the women and girls.

An added problem is that most current diagnostic assessments do not consider sex differences and only give examples of the male profile of behaviour. The knowledge and experience of an enlightened clinician are essential in both asking the right questions and interpreting the data to provide an accurate outcome.

The remaining chapters cover all aspects of life from childhood through to adolescence and adulthood. Each stage in a woman's life brings new problems and dilemmas. The experiences described by those who participated in the author's research demonstrate how the girls and women had a rotten time in their school years through a lack of diagnosis and appropriate understanding and support.

Developing appropriate approaches will maximise the positive and minimise the negative elements of the women's journey through life.

The question is posed as to the value of a diagnosis in adulthood. Women often shared the same sense of relief and self-acceptance as men but to an even greater degree. The diagnosis provided an explanation of the problems they had experienced throughout their lives and now they could be themselves without hiding their problems. The descriptions throughout the book demonstrate the extraordinary resilience shown by these women, particularly in their compensatory strategies. These efforts often come at a price; exhaustion, breakdown and mental health issues are commonly mentioned by these women. It cannot be stressed enough that the ill-effects are the consequence of living with autism, not the conditions or symptoms, which may be considered in isolation. This is a very important point for clinicians.

Throughout the book, all phases of life are touched on and the message is that life is hard for everyone, particularly in regard to personal relationships, sexuality, gender identity, pregnancy and parenting, health and well-being and employment, but is even harder for those on the autism spectrum. The chapters on these aspects of life are encouraging, giving useful tips and reflecting that we can all be different and that this is to be celebrated.

The chapter 'Ageing with Autism' is important as there are many women in their later years who have only recently received a diagnosis. It is important to say that it is never too late to gain an understanding of your life. In the final chapter, the most relevant quote is: 'The first step is for professionals to understand that the profile shows itself differently in females than males. You have to work a bit harder to find it, but it's there. And just because it's not too visible, doesn't mean it's not "severe".'

This book endorses my clinical experiences of working with females on the autism spectrum and validates the importance of diagnosis at any time in a person's life. I highly recommend this book for all professionals involved in diagnosis and in supporting girls and women on the autism spectrum.

Dr Judith Gould
Consultant Clinical Psychologist and Director,
The Lorna Wing Centre for Autism

Acknowledgements

My thanks go to the following people, without whom this book wouldn't exist; Jess, my daughter and professional protector from the world of people, for looking after the women who contributed. 'Dr' Chris Girvan for proofreading and access to research papers, because he's a proper academic and I'm not. Dr Becky Heaver for having the right sort of autism to love formatting reference lists. (Imposter? I don't think so.) My big brother, Frank, for pedanticism. Sarah F. at ASSERT (Brighton and Hove) for stats and musings. Professor Tony Attwood and Dr Judith Gould for their gracious answering of questions.

I am indebted to the women with autism and the families of girls with autism who took the time to participate by answering my endless questions; and also to those who retweeted and shared my requests for help. In total, the first-hand experiences of over 30 girls and women with autism have been included, along with academic research, my professional and personal experiences and those of other authors – both those with Autism Spectrum Disorder (ASD) and practitioners in the field. Some prefer to remain anonymous; others who personally and/or professionally contributed are listed here at their request: Jen Leavesley, Heidi M. Sands, Melanie Peekes, Susan Nairn, Dr Catriona Stewart, Scottish Women with Autism Network (SWAN), Kathleen Comber, Lynda Anderson, Becky Heaver, Kim Richardson, Helen Ellis, Jemimah Pearce, Judith Vaughan, Anna Vaughan, C. Linsky, Emma Dalrymple, Allison Palmer, Claire Robinson, Debbie Allan, Darci, Rose Way, Rachel Sloan, Jade Walker, Makayla Maddison, Anya K. Ustaszewski.

Preface

Why?

My son was the last in my family to undergo diagnosis for autism, a couple of years after I had received mine (a long story for another day). At the appointment, I gave our family history to the psychiatrist carrying out the diagnostic assessment. I included details of my own autism diagnosis and those of other members of our family to give some context of an inherited condition. The psychiatrist questioned my diagnosis, asking who had diagnosed me. He asked how I could have autism because I didn't look like I had autism and I was having a two-way conversation with him. I replied that maybe it's because I'm an adult and a woman. He looked at me incredulously and said, with obvious contempt: 'Are you trying to tell me that being a woman makes a difference?' I replied (sigh) that it did. He shook his head in disbelief.

I was furious and sad that the person responsible for my son's (and someone else's daughter's) diagnosis was ignorant and frankly disrespectful. I knew there was nothing I could say. I shut up and hoped that we could just continue with what we had come for. I waited until we had left the room before I cried and exploded with frustration. I wish this was the only occasion where I have had to justify my diagnosis because I don't look autistic enough, but it isn't and it won't be.

If the gatekeepers of diagnosis and subsequent support are unaware, individuals and families will be powerless to get what they need. The injustice of this makes me unbelievably angry.

This is why I wrote this book.

Introduction

Just because you can't see it doesn't mean it's not there.

Since the beginning of our modern-day understanding of autism, the general consensus has been that there are substantially more males with the condition than there are females. Until fairly recently, this has been largely accepted as fact. I frequently discuss this with people attending the training courses that I deliver, and the overwhelming opinion is that more males than females have autism and 'that's just the way it is'. Others express surprise that women can have autism at all. We still have a way to go to educate some people as to the real picture, partly because we don't know what the real picture looks like yet – but we're getting there.

Increasingly, the questioning of the origin of this 'fact' and the subsequent examination of potential explanations have given rise to a new understanding: that is, there are plenty of women with autism, but we just hide it better, make sense of it differently or present it in a way that slips under the radar of those looking for classic (male) indicators derived from the (almost) exclusively male research (or at least research that does not differentiate according to gender).

I am one of those women with autism who has hidden it extremely well, to the point that I couldn't even see it myself. I say 'hidden', although this was not a conscious ploy – more a subconscious response to a life-long understanding that the 'real me' was not usually particularly welcome or approved of by others around me. I wanted to get by with the minimum of hassle and I didn't want to stick out for the wrong reasons. Therefore, I used my rather capable brain to work out how to do that with relative success (despite considerable harm to myself mentally and physically) and kept 'real me' out of sight as often as possible. Real me only leaks out when the rote-learning system I have devised has insufficient data to maintain the facade. Real me is also allowed out in times of complete comfort and acceptance (it takes a rare soul to love and accept without judgement a squeaking, rocking and clapping adult woman – thank you, thank you, thank you, Keith).

I was diagnosed with autism at the age of 43 years. At this point in my life I had been working exclusively in the field of autism for five years, both as an employee and more recently as a self-employed person running my own training organisation, Hendrickx Associates (www.asperger-training.com). I had completed a Master's degree in autism, written five books on autism, spoken at many conferences, trained several thousand practitioners in autism and worked with well over a hundred individuals with autism. It seems ludicrous even to me that someone so immersed in both the theory and practice of autism could not 'spot' it in herself.

The reason that it took me so long to do so was that I was guilty of doing exactly the same thing that everyone else had been doing to women with autism for all these years: I was comparing myself with the male presentation, and I didn't fit. Specifically, I was using my partner, Keith, who has an Autism Spectrum Disorder (ASD) diagnosis himself, as my control sample. In fact, I was so convinced of my somewhat neurotypical (NT) status that Keith and I wrote a book about our Asperger Syndrome (AS)/NT relationship (Hendrickx and Newton 2007). Increasingly, I realised that we were very similar in many ways and that I just 'got' him in a way that other NT people had struggled to do. I realised how incredibly logical, routine-orientated and systematic I am, but with no interest in technical things like he has. My fascination is people and how they operate (most typically articulated by a frown and 'Why do they do that?'). I realised that I struggle enormously socially, yet do social events anyway at great mental cost to myself, because I am supposed to, whereas he will just say 'no' and avoid any discomfort.

For several years, my analytical, self-obsessed nature was having a ball trying to work out this paradox. The realisation and the answer came slowly and steadily every time I met a woman with autism through my work as an ASD specialist and coach. I would work with someone professionally and, on hearing their life stories and their way of being, I was frequently shocked by the similarity between their lives and my own. Numerous failed relationships, failed jobs, many jettisoned, short-lived projects where interest disappeared overnight, anxiety, 'madness' (to quote numerous people in my own life) – it was all so familiar. I could see precisely how these things fitted the diagnostic criteria and I was able to begin applying that understanding to myself. After a few more years of data-gathering and self-analysis, I went for a diagnosis and my suspicions were unreservedly confirmed.

Conversely, I felt that working in the field of autism made it harder for me to 'come out'. I was certainly not ashamed or in denial; my favourite people (and most of my family) have autism. The fact was, I had been surrounded by it and yet hadn't realised I had it myself. To the uninitiated that must sound very strange, less so perhaps to those in the field. Along with this, my outward presentation is deliberately extremely well constructed. My life-long special interest in studying people has both served me well and also shot me in the foot: I don't look like someone who cannot cope with simple everyday interactions or instructions. The aim of this life's work of mine has been to learn how to be invisible and never appear less than 100 per cent perfect and capable. Phew! But it is a mighty and foolish bar to set. The prospect of disclosure and admitting to actually being different and (in my eyes) less than the perfectly acceptable person I have always striven to be, was a huge personal dilemma. I have never considered any other person with autism as inadequate, but my own logic results in me applying these ridiculous standards to myself (black-and-white perfectionism – it's all in the diagnostic criteria). I am also fully aware of the level of discrimination that people with autism experience and felt that professional disclosure could affect my work and how people treat me. In my experience, once someone knows, they look at you differently, they treat you differently; and my goal has always been to be invisible. So at the same time as occasionally supporting recently diagnosed individuals on a professional basis, I was coming to terms with my own diagnosis and what this meant for me psychologically and practically.

It took me three years following my diagnosis to tell anyone beyond my immediate family. The response, both personally and professionally, has been overwhelmingly positive, but the dichotomy of being both visible and striving to be invisible remains. Forty-six years of trying to perfect the 'normal' persona is difficult to drop, although increasingly I'm getting too tired to maintain the pretence and self-acceptance is getting a little easier. My personal journey as a person with autism continues every minute of every day. The knowing is just the start; the understanding and the living with it never ends. Almost every day I learn new things that make sense of decades of confusion. I believe that the only people I have ever met who truly 'get it' are other people with autism. It's just how it is; you cannot truly imagine an experience of life that you can't see and have never had. Despite that, the need to let other people into our world, to help them to try to 'get it', is important and the quest continues.

As I said earlier, knowledge of the way life is experienced by women on the autism spectrum is relatively new and, as yet, poorly understood. What I wanted this book to achieve was to combine existing research and knowledge with my own personal experiences and those of a number of women with autism and the families of girls with autism. I wanted to compile a view of life as a female with autism from beginning to end in all its glory!

I am not suggesting for one moment that this is a definitive picture of life for all women with autism; it is a small sample from a large and varied community designed to broaden understanding and, I hope, offer support. It is the best I could do and I hope it's OK. I hope the inclusion of my own experiences does not appear self-indulgent; I just wanted to provide as much first-hand insight as I could within my limited resources. My experience is, of course, no more representative than anyone else's. We're all different; yet all the same.

I hope that through this work professionals will consider new indicators to watch out for and will ask different questions when making those initial diagnoses; also, that practitioners will see past the invisible persona presentation and not disbelieve; and that women who suspect they may have an ASD will find solidarity, shared experiences and the courage to seek diagnosis if that is what they need. Many highly esteemed professionals in the world of autism are writing about, talking about and researching the idea that gender does matter when considering a diagnosis, profile and support. I hope to share their work and add a little of my own to the conversation.

This book does not seek to detract from the male or non-gender-specific experience of ASD, but rather to present the missing piece of the partial picture that has been in the public domain for many years. Gender makes a difference. Pretty much all of the initial research into autism was carried out on boys, and their profile was deemed to be the default, so it is not surprising that girls never got much of a look in. Gender was never considered an issue; but it is. The girls are being missed now due to them being overlooked in the first place. And the girls need to know who they are.

For information

This book assumes the reader has some basic knowledge of ASD and its characteristics. I have not gone into detail with regard to theoretical concepts and behaviours, beyond those that are specifically relevant to females. There are many other superb publications by well-respected authors who have done this. Characteristics presented may be indicative of autism, but may also, when considered in isolation, be caused by something else. The inclusion of characteristics does not imply that ASD is the only explanation for them. This book does not give the reader the knowledge or experience to make a diagnosis of ASD and should be used in conjunction with expert advice and assessment.

This book discusses females with ASD right across the autism spectrum and has attempted to include perspectives of individuals (and their families) affected by autism with associated learning disabilities, although that number has sadly been smaller than I would have liked. The anonymous verbatim quotes used throughout the book come from a group of women with autism and parents of girls with autism who agreed to contribute. They all contributed via emailed questionnaires during 2014 on a variety of topics as covered in the chapters. In total, over 30 women shared their experiences. Some contributed more and/or different information than others due to age, specific life experiences (i.e. whether they were parents or had experience of employment). Most of the women were from the UK, with some from the USA and elsewhere in Europe. Age ranged from 5 year to 62 years. Age of diagnosis ranged from 4 years to 56 years.

Some chapters of this book (e.g., those to do with employment and relationships) may have more relevance to those without significant learning disability and a greater expectation of independence (i.e. individuals with Asperger Syndrome). In some parts of the book there is greater emphasis on more intellectually able females with ASD.

The term 'Autism Spectrum Disorder' (ASD) is used throughout to reflect the *Diagnostic and Statistical Manual of Mental Disorders Fifth Edition* (DSM-5, American Psychiatric Association 2013) specification and to encompass all forms of autism. This is the publisher's preferred term of reference. 'Neurotypical' (NT) is used as a term to describe those not on the autism spectrum and with a neurologically typical profile. It is a standard term used for ease, not to homogenise any group. Within quoted contributor and reference responses, terms such as 'Aspie', 'Asperger Syndrome' and 'high-functioning autism' are used. These are the writers' own words. I use the term 'challenging behaviour' in inverted commas as this is a phrase in common usage by both professionals and families, and so is useful to succinctly explain a concept of behaviour that is considered to be a challenge for others, but one that I feel is often used incorrectly. I have a personal dislike for the terms 'high-functioning', 'low-functioning', 'mild' and 'severe' to indicate how a person's autism affects them, for reasons I will not go into here other than to say that they are, in my opinion, usually poorly understood, misused and therefore often misleading and unhelpful. If I have used any of these terms in this book, they will either be qualified and specific in definition, or will be other people's terminology that I am quoting or referencing. The same principle applies to terms such as 'deficit', 'wrong', 'amiss' or 'abnormal' – this is the researchers' or participants' terminology that is being reproduced, not my own perspective. If some quotes appear negative, this is to provide a broad view of different perspectives of autism along with the thoughts and terminology of those affected, rather than any personal opinion of my own. I am not promoting negativity about autism or those affected by it, nor am I presenting only a rosy view.

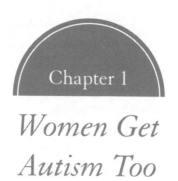

Women Get Autism Too

The findings suggest that we should not assume that everything found in males with autism applies to females. This is an important example of the diversity within the 'spectrum'.

DR MENG-CHUAN LAI, AUTISM RESEARCH
CENTRE (UNIVERSITY OF CAMBRIDGE 2013)

Gender differences in autism – research review

Autism Spectrum Disorder (ASD) is a broad, complex and still, apparently, relatively unfathomable condition, although our knowledge and understanding about it are constantly increasing. Recent data from the Centers for Disease Control and Prevention in the US suggest that 1 in 68 people have an ASD (Autism and Developmental Disabilities Monitoring Network 2014). We are learning that autism is a more diverse disorder than was originally described by Dr Kanner more than 70 years ago. Yet despite all the recent breakthroughs in research, we still can't explain it fully; we're not even close. We know even less about whether and/or how gender affects individuals with ASD. Research that investigates and differentiates the male and female profile, presentation and experience of autism is fairly scarce, thereby perpetuating the myth that autism is a significantly male-dominated condition, or alternatively that gender is simply not a consideration.

Although the development of the diagnostic profile was based almost entirely on a male phenotype (Kopp and Gillberg 1992), it is important to note that mention was made of differences in the presentation of female autism by both Leo Kanner and Hans Asperger in the 1940s – perhaps it was not considered to be significant at the time. Kanner (1943) had noted that one girl did not understand games and pretended to be a dog, walking on all fours and making dog noises. Despite evidence that suggests that male and female brains in the general population have a different neurological profile (McCarthy *et al.* 2012; Ruigrok *et al.* 2014), it appears that researchers have hitherto thought that autism somehow overrides these differences and rather than having the neurological physiology and cognitive profile of a 'man' or 'woman', one is simply 'autistic'. Personally, I think this unlikely, but this is how it has largely been viewed until fairly recently.

There appear to be several threads for discussion here, which current research has investigated to some degree:

- Is there a measurable and/or observable difference – biologically, neurologically, behaviourally and/or cognitively – between males and females with autism?

- How does that difference manifest cognitively and behaviourally?

- Do the current diagnostic criteria take into account any identified differences and accurately identify and diagnose males and females with autism?

- If not, is there potential for under-diagnosis of females?

- What do we need to do about any different manifestation in terms of diagnostic tools, diagnostic understanding and support?

Due to the paucity of women diagnosed with autism, it is difficult to find sufficient numbers of age- and developmentally matched females to participate in research that might show significant findings (Mandy *et al.* 2012). Put simply, if girls are not getting diagnosed because the criteria do not pick them up (because they weren't considered in the creation of the criteria), there will be fewer diagnosed and included in research; research will therefore draw conclusions from smaller samples of the females who do match the male criteria…and on it goes…

Many esteemed individuals working in the autism field have commented and considered female ASD as worthy of differentiation from the standard profile; they include Tony Attwood, Simon Baron-Cohen, Svenny Kopp, Lorna Wing and Judith Gould, all of whom have put their substantial professional weight behind acknowledging and improving understanding and diagnosis for women on the autism spectrum. Practitioners are gathering data and developing lists of characteristics seen in women and girls (Marshall 2014). But a broader academic knowledge-base is thin on the ground. In contrast, the autobiographical and anecdotal published works on autism have a plethora of women with autism as contributors: Temple Grandin, Liane Holliday Willey, Wenn Lawson (formerly Wendy Lawson), Rudy Simone and Donna Williams, to name but a few. It seems that the women themselves have the words and the desire to speak out about their lives, but the 'experts' are not doing so to the same degree on their behalf in a scientific or practitioner context. These women are well-known names and faces in the autism world – confident public speakers and educators, sharing their unique perspective – but until now they have been considered largely indistinguishable from the men.

There are several different views that are worthy of consideration when discussing the male–female autism issue (Lai *et al.* 2011). One is that male and female autism may differ on a neurological and/or cognitive level (Carter *et al.* 2007). Another suggests that perhaps there are fewer females with autism because they are somehow protected against developing the condition (Jacquemont *et al.* 2014; Volkmar, Szatmari and Sparrow 1993), which may also explain why many neurodevelopmental conditions appear to affect more males than females (Zahn-Waxler, Shirtcliff and Marceau 2008). We also have to consider that the tools used for identifying autism may have a male gender bias and therefore are not 'picking up' female autism if it has a distinctly separate behavioural quality. ASDs are currently diagnosed behaviourally and observationally, therefore despite any potential similarities or differences on a cognitive or neurodevelopmental level, it may simply be that females present their autism differently through behaviours that are not included in the current diagnostic criteria (Kopp and Gillberg 1992). If this is the case, it is likely that clinicians making diagnoses need to view the current criteria more broadly to ensure that female behaviour is considered. More importantly, it may be necessary to develop a new set of diagnostic criteria that fully includes the female presentation of autism. More on this subject in Chapter 17.

Sex ratios

There is huge variation in estimations of sex ratios within autism. Wing (1981) found a 2.6:1 male to female ratio in a study of children in one London borough in the 1970s, but these were children with low IQ and it is commonly believed that more females with autism exist within this intellectual bracket than within higher IQ levels (Volkmar *et al.* 1993). In a review of 37 epidemiological studies spanning the years from 1966 to 2005, Fombonne (2005) found male to female ratios ranging from 1.4:1 to 15.7:1. Tony Attwood (2007) carried out an analysis of over 100 diagnostic assessments in his clinic over 12 years and found a 4:1 male to female ratio. In two Brighton-based adult autism support services, the male to female ratios are 2:1 and 3:1. This vast range simply means that we don't really know. There are many factors involved in research and practice that may influence ratios, including diagnostic criteria, referrer beliefs about autism, clinician assessment, sample size and type, and IQ. What is generally accepted is that women and girls at the higher IQ end of autism are falling through the net and there are therefore likely to be more females with an ASD than are currently diagnosed.

It has been found that girls were significantly less likely to receive an autism spectrum diagnosis than boys, even when their symptoms were equally severe (Russell, Steer and Golding 2011), perhaps due to gender expectations and stereotyping by parents and professionals. Theories such as the 'extreme male brain theory' (Baron-Cohen 2002) may also have contributed to the popular view of autism as a 'male' condition, which may influence professionals in their consideration of autism as a likely diagnosis for a female.

Neurological profile

While sex differences in autism have been largely ignored (Bölte *et al.* 2011), there is a small amount of work that has considered neurological perspectives of differences in brain development and functioning as potential factors in explaining male and female autism. Lai *et al.* (2013) found that aspects of brain neuro-anatomy are sex dependent. Furthermore, this study also found minimal overlap between the neuro-anatomical features of males and females with autism, suggesting that males and females with autism may actually be neurally and cognitively distinct. Craig *et al.* (2007) found differences in the density of grey and white matter in areas of the brain linked to social behaviour deficits.

For some time there has been a general view that females with autism are somehow more impaired than males with autism and that perhaps the neural or cognitive 'damage' that has to occur in order for a female to get autism needs to be greater than for a male. One study found that girls with 'high-functioning' autism who attended a clinic were 'more neuro-cognitively affected' (Nyden, Hjelmquist and Gilberg 2000, p.185) than boys with the same diagnosis attending the same clinic. The girls were seen to have more 'extensive deficits' in theory of mind and executive functioning than the boys. The study suggests that girls attending the clinic may be in greater need of support than the boys (Nyden *et al.* 2000). Volkmar *et al.* (1993) found that in IQ testing, larger numbers of females with autism were at the lower end of the IQ scale and had learning disabilities than males, which appears to support the suggestion above that in general autism needs to be 'worse' for it to manifest in women, with fewer women appearing in the intellectually higher-functioning category of autism. Other work has similar findings (Lord, Schopler and Revicki 1982; Tsai and Beisler 1983; Wing 1981).

One of the most powerful theories in autism, which has had an impact on both public perception and sex differences, is the work of Professor Simon Baron-Cohen and other researchers from the Autism Research Centre in Cambridge, UK, and relates to levels of testosterone, androgen and other neurobiologically occurring chemicals. Several studies focus on the 'extreme male brain theory' of autism developed by Baron-Cohen (2002) and how this manifests in women. Baron-Cohen's original work did not largely differentiate between males and females with autism, but he and others have since taken this further. The concept of masculinised behaviour in females with autism is one of the more researched areas in gender difference, which has had mixed reactions from the autism community. According to androgen theory of autism (Ingudomnukul *et al.* 2007), autism is partly caused by elevated foetal testosterone levels. These levels are correlated both positively and inversely with a number of autistic characteristics, including eye contact, vocabulary and social relationships. Further research revisiting these ideas (Bejerot *et al.* 2012) confirms that testosterone levels in women with autism were higher than control samples and that these women displayed more masculinised characteristics. It also found that men with autism presented more feminised characteristics, indicating that rather than women with autism being more masculinised *per se*, both genders may be more androgynous and represent a 'gender defiant disorder' (Bejerot *et al.* 2012, p.9). They go on to suggest that, 'gender incoherence in individuals with ASD is to be expected and should be regarded as one reflection of the wide autism phenotype' (Bejerot *et al.* 2012, p.9). The notion that females with autism present a profile – physically, cognitively and/or behaviourally – less stereotypically feminised than that of neurotypical (NT) females is one that will be explored more fully in other chapters of this book as it is something recognised anecdotally by many women with autism I have met. The 'tomboy' is recognised as a potential diagnostic indicator, although not all women with autism fit this profile.

Behavioural manifestation

There has not been a great deal of research into gender-differentiated behaviour manifestation, and certainly no large-scale studies (Giarelli *et al.* 2010). Anecdotally, as we will see later in this book, professional and personal accounts testify to distinct differences in visible presentation between males and females with autism, but this has not been quantified or discussed formally to any great degree. Research that has taken place so far has focused on very specific elements of the current diagnostic criteria when comparing gender performance. I have outlined a few studies below by way of illustration. Available research in this area is very hard to find, simply because it is scarce.

Knickmeyer, Wheelwright and Baron-Cohen (2008) examined sex-typical play in girls with autism. Their research found that girls with autism did not show a preference for female-typical items when engaged in play that did not involve pretence. This may show evidence of the hypothesis of masculinisation in girls with autism; alternatively, the researchers suggest these girls may be less susceptible to social factors that influence toy selection by girls and boys. However, if this were the case, we may have expected them to find the same lack of preference for gender-based non-pretence toys in boys with autism, but this was not the case; boys showed a preference for sex-typical non-pretence toys. When looking at games that did involve pretence (imagination), boys with autism showed virtually no interest, whereas girls with autism were very much engaged in imaginary play, as per typically developing girls. Imagination, usually considered to be an area of difficulty in individuals with autism, may not be affected in the same way in girls as it is in boys, with girls often retreating into fantasy worlds as respite from the stress of being in the real one. The Knickmeyer *et al.* (2008) study also cites research that suggests that pretence may be a skill that is developed via nurture more in girls than in boys: parent–daughter pretence play is more likely than parent–son pretence play.

Another study looked specifically at one element of behaviour and compared response inhibition in males and females with autism (Lemon *et al.* 2011). Individuals were asked to respond to a light being switched on by pressing a button as quickly as possible. The study found that females with autism were significantly slower to *stop* responding (i.e. to inhibit their responses) than either males with autism or NT males and females. Males with autism did not show any difference in response inhibition times to NT males and females. This study only focuses on one small area of behaviour, but may suggest that females with autism have a different neurobehavioural profile to males with autism. The consequences of impaired inhibitory control include impulsiveness, risk-taking and general executive dysfunction, including planning and decision-making. This may also impact on other social difficulties, such as appropriate behavioural responses, particularly when under stress (Lemon *et al.* 2011).

Carter *et al.* (2007) looked at sex differences in toddlers with autism and found that girls scored more highly in visual reception than boys, while boys scored more highly in language, motor and social competence than girls. They report statistically significant cognitive and development profile differences between girls and boys with autism aged 1–3 years. A study of a similar age group (Hartley and Sikora 2009) found many parallels in the male and female profile, but some 'subtle but potentially important differences between the male and female ASD phenotype' (p.179). Boys showed more repetitive, restricted behaviours than girls, and girls showed more communication deficits, sleep problems and anxiety. When looking at an older age group (3–18 years), teachers reported that males with autism externalise their social problems more readily than females and therefore are more likely to be identified as needing support in the classroom (Mandy *et al.* 2012). This work also agreed with Hartley and Sikora (2009) that there were subtle differences between the sexes. They found that girls had more 'emotional problems' (Mandy *et al.* 2012, p.1310) and better fine motor skills. As with other studies, restricted, repetitive behaviour was seen less in girls than in boys.

Bölte *et al.* (2011) found that executive functioning was scored more highly by girls with autism, and attention to detail was scored more highly in boys with autism. This may add weight to the suggestion that boys with autism show more stereotypical ritualised behaviours than girls with autism (Carter *et al.* 2007). It may also support the idea that women with autism have more 'life events' than men with autism (van Wijngaarden-Cremers 2012) as their better executive functioning may enable them to be more active in life in general (this does not mean that their decision-making is always effective).

Rather than the 'extreme autistic aloneness' personality mentioned by Kanner (1943, p.242), Kopp and Gillberg (1992) saw girls in their study being more 'clinging' (p.96) to others, imitating their speech and movements without a deeper understanding of the silent laws of ordinary social interaction. They also saw more repetitive questioning and 'almost constant use of language' (p.97), which is not commonly expected in the typical (male) profile of autism. This verbosity can appear social and interactive, but may be, on examination, scripted, learned or largely self-centric in nature. Comments on females' ability to appear socially typical and mask their autistic behaviours occur in the literature time and time again (Attwood 2007; Gould and Ashton-Smith 2011; Lai *et al.* 2011), but as yet, only a few professionals in the field are acting on this to improve the situation by changing diagnostic processes. Kopp and Gillberg's (2011) later work found that the following behaviours were much more typical of girls with autism than boys: 'avoids demands', 'very determined', 'careless with physical appearance' and 'interacts mostly with younger children' (pp.2881–2882).

Lai *et al.* (2011) found that on comparing boys and girls with autism, both were 'equally autistic' (p.5) as children, but that as adults the females showed fewer social communication difficulties, suggesting that they may have learned compensatory strategies and may be more motivated to do so throughout their lives in order to appear more 'socially typical' (p.6). The men in this study had not followed the same trajectory into adulthood. This masking of autistic characteristics has been documented by others in the field (Attwood 2007; Gould and Ashton-Smith 2011) and will be discussed in much greater detail throughout this book. It is suggested that women with autism are able to apply the systematic nature of their autistic brain (Baron-Cohen 2002) to the study and replication of people skills in order to imitate and participate socially. However, the mechanical (rather than intuitive) basis of these strategies means that at times of stress, in unexpected situations or after a period of time, it may be impossible for them to be maintained (Lai *et al.* 2011). For some women this can mean that they present a very capable front that cannot be maintained beyond certain limits, after which it collapses (and sometimes so does she). What has not yet been measured is the toll that this socially typical facade takes on the individual over a period of time.

It has also been suggested that women with autism are better at masking their autistic features due to better self-awareness and self-referential abilities (Attwood 2007; Lai *et al.* 2011). This increased ability would support women's reported improved understanding of what is required socially and how to meet these expectations. Self-reporting of autistic characteristics was also seen to be higher in women, despite fewer behaviours being observed when tested with clinical autism diagnostic tools (ADOs). This suggests that despite less obvious observable characteristics, women have the same (if not higher) perception of their autism, and its impact, as men. In relation to this, it has been suggested that in studies that require parent observation and evaluation of autistic characteristics, parents may have higher expectations of the social and communication behaviour of girls than they do of boys, which may skew any findings (McLennan, Lord and Schopler 1993).

Chapter 2

Considering Autism Spectrum Disorder in Females

Many women whom I support have little or no faith in the mental health system due to very bad experiences. It is interesting that many women had to make the suggestion of autism to their clinicians in order for it to be pursued, rather than the clinicians noticing their autistic traits.

ASD SPECIALIST SUPPORT WORKER (2014)

Getting a diagnosis

Until recently, commonly used diagnostic criteria, such as the *Diagnostic and Statistical Manual of Mental Disorders* (DSM) and International Classification of Diseases (ICD), have not considered sex differences at all (Gould and Ashton-Smith 2011; Lord *et al.* 1982). The updated DSM-5 criteria (American Psychiatric Association 2013) show significant changes to the general criteria for Autism Spectrum Disorders (ASDs) with the removal of independent diagnosis for Asperger Syndrome and other changes to the required indicators. Also, there is mention of sex differences for the first time: 'In clinic samples females tend to be more likely to show accompanying intellectual disability, which suggests that girls without accompanying intellectual disability or language delays may go unrecognized, perhaps because of subtler manifestation of social and communication difficulties.' (American Psychiatric Association 2013). Mandy (2013) adds his own comment on the potential implications of this:

In this sense, the architects of the DSM-5 have laid down a challenge to researchers: Provide an account of the female phenotype, so that clinicians can learn to better identify, and help, females on the autism spectrum [without an accompanying intellectual disability]. (Mandy 2013)

The DSM-5 also includes the following new specifier, which may assist the female cause: 'C. Symptoms must be present in the early development period (but may not become fully manifest until social demands exceed limited capacities, or may be masked by learned strategies in later life' (American Psychiatric Association 2013).

The explicit recognition that autism may not be 'fully manifest' until life becomes unmanageable for an individual will, it is to be hoped, aid those seeking adult diagnosis who may, up until now, have been told: 'You can't have autism; you would have been diagnosed by now if you did'. Furthermore, the assertion that 'learned strategies' may be adopted, and the inference that they should be considered as part of the evidence of potentially autistic indicators, should aid more accurate diagnosis in both males and females, but may have particular relevance to the documented masking abilities of females.

The new DSM-5 criteria place a greater emphasis on restricted, stereotyped behaviours being observed, yet some research has found that females with ASD do not exhibit these behaviours to the same degree as males, or at least not in the same way, which may exclude some females from receiving a diagnosis of ASD (Mandy *et al.* 2012). Some autism research professionals do not feel that non-gender-specific criteria are necessarily in need of changing to better identify autism in females, but that the onus must be on clinicians to interpret them accurately with a good understanding of how autism may present in females. When training clinicians to use the Diagnostic Interview for Social and Communication Disorders (DISCO) assessment tool, Dr Judith Gould encourages clinicians to examine the data gathered with a broader view:

The criteria relate to the condition which are not gender specific. The point is how do clinicians interpret the criteria rather than changing the criteria? [...] The key is asking the right questions and sadly that only comes from experience and knowledge about the female presentation of the condition. Educating professionals as we do in our diagnostic training is one of the ways forward. (Gould 2014)

Current diagnostic tests and tools do not consider sex differences and only follow the diagnostic requirements as laid down by the DSM criteria. Frazier (2014) suggests that sex-specific norms for some diagnostic processes might be helpful. The teaching of these methods should provide gender-differentiated examples to give new clinicians the breadth of the presentation of the autistic profile. This book attempts to do the same by providing first-hand and professional examples of how autism shows itself in and affects females.

The diagnostic process itself takes on a number of forms depending on the age and/or intellectual ability of the individual and the culture of the diagnostic service or clinician. There is no definitive test for autism and no standard way of carrying out an assessment. The outcome of the diagnostic assessment has a subjective element and is based on the quality and quantity of evidence gathered and the experience and opinion of the clinician or clinicians involved. This explains why the knowledge and experience of the clinician are essential both in asking the right questions to elicit the necessary data and in interpreting that data to provide an accurate outcome – processes that are particularly relevant in the case of females. Eileen Riley-Hall (2012) provides a detailed account of the diagnostic process (in the US) that she went through with her two daughters. Following the diagnosis, professionals should have good knowledge of local referral points for services and links to information about understanding the diagnosis for both the individual and their family members. Diagnosis is only the beginning of the journey, not the end.

As previously mentioned, females are significantly less likely to receive a diagnosis than males (Giarelli *et al.* 2010; Russell *et al.* 2011), and by using current diagnostic methods, some females may 'look' less autistic, but not actually 'be' or 'feel' any less autistic (Lai *et al.* 2011). Girls and boys may be identified for diagnostic assessment at a similar age, but boys are more likely to receive an autism diagnosis whereas girls may receive a different diagnosis despite both sexes displaying markers/signs clinically associated with autism (Giarelli *et al.* 2010). It may be that clinicians who are expecting autism to be more common in males are attributing certain behaviours to autism in boys and attributing the same behaviours to different conditions in girls. Equally, it may be that clinicians are expecting males and females with autism to behave in the same way, even though boys' and girls' behaviour is not considered to be identical in the typically developing population (McCarthy *et al.* 2012; Ruigrok *et al.* 2014). Head, McGillivray and Stokes (2014) studied social and emotional skills in males and females with autism and compared them to those in typically developing peers aged 12–16 years. They found that females with autism scored higher than males with autism, and at a similar level to typically developing males, but lower than typically developing females. They concluded that this could partly explain the potential under-diagnosis of females as social presentation is not currently gender-differentiated in the diagnostic criteria. They suggest that if a female with autism presents as more highly functioning than a male with autism, their abilities may appear superficially typical (and similar to that of a typical male) and therefore not be considered as notable if the clinician is using the male autistic social skills profile.

In children without an autism diagnosis, it is more common for girls to receive diagnoses of general developmental delay or seizure disorder – staring spells and seizure-like activity were five times more commonly diagnosed in girls than in boys (Giarelli *et al.* 2010). Kopp and Gillberg (1992) report seeing many girls in their centre who 'do not clinically present the picture usually associated with autistic disorder' (p.90). These girls fulfil the criteria in childhood, but as they mature they present a considerably different profile to their male counterparts. Kopp and Gillberg (1992) suggest that some clinicians do not believe that these adult women could ever have fitted the full autistic profile earlier in life. A potential factor in these girls not presenting sufficiently to receive a positive diagnosis may be that the diagnostic criteria do not require responses to be made within a given time-frame. One of the noted issues for girls with autism is the length of time it takes them to respond socially – they may get there in the end, but are noticeably slower than same-age peers (Nichols, Moravcik and Tetenbaum 2009). Clinicians' attention can be diverted by the presentation of other co-morbid mental health conditions in teenage and adult life – conditions such as anorexia and anxiety disorders, which may be part of the autism profile but may not lead automatically to considering autism as the causal factor (Kopp and Gillberg 1992; Simone 2010). W. Lawson (1998) describes how it took 25 years to be diagnosed with Asperger Syndrome after being wrongly diagnosed with schizophrenia. The majority of the women participants questioned for this book had experienced years of mental health difficulties (mainly anxiety) and interventions before receiving an autism diagnosis.

> [It took] five years or so to finally pinpoint the condition after I scored highly positive in a preliminary written questionnaire regarding AS [Asperger Syndrome]. The difficulty came in my other issues obfuscating the root cause of my behaviourisms. I've been called anywhere from bipolar to schizophrenic and have had medication provided thusly to combat those symptoms. (Woman with autism)

> I have been misdiagnosed most of my life, including hearing doctors tell my mother that I had emotional problems, that I was trying to get attention, that I had nervous problems or that I was neurotic. Later I was diagnosed with learning disabilities in high school. In college, a doctor who initially thought I was psychotic eventually diagnosed me as having Severe Neurosis with Schizoid tendencies. (Woman with autism)

Nichols *et al.* (2009) suggest that routes to eventual autism diagnosis for a female can include the following steps, and that a fuller knowledge and understanding of these can aid the clinician in considering autism when assessing the person and can potentially facilitate more accurate diagnosis:

- Previous diagnosis of another disorder or several disorders, including Attention Deficit Hyperactivity Disorder (ADHD), anxiety, depression, obsessive-compulsive disorder, eating disorder. Nichols *et al.* suggest that the older the girl, the more diagnoses she is likely to have collected.

- A diagnosis of social anxiety or general difficulty in social situations.

- Adult women with a previous diagnosis of schizophrenia or psychotic disorder.

- Another family member has an ASD diagnosis.

- Presentation or apparent deterioration of capacity to cope as adolescence approaches, where social relationships become more nuanced and complex.

- In adolescence, girls may not demonstrate typically 'female' social interests, such as fashion and relationships.

The process of change for the individual begins with diagnostic measures and how clinicians are implementing them. If the tools are not accurate in identifying girls, then clinicians will have a hard job accurately assessing them. It has been suggested that sex-specific behavioural or cognitive autism diagnostic criteria may be necessary to accurately reflect the true sex ratio (e.g., Lai *et al.* 2011). Until the time when new criteria are developed that encompass female ASD, clinicians will have to fill in the gaps themselves, by developing a broader understanding of what to look for and who to listen to. Tony Attwood has developed a Screening Test for parents to support identification of girls with autism (Attwood 2013). The questions focus on specifically female presentations of autism, such as gender toy preference, fantasy worlds and relationships with both people and animals. The test is used as part of a broader diagnostic assessment and at least begins to ask the right questions of parents in order to build a more accurate female profile. Marshall (2014) has developed (and continues to do so) a list of characteristics commonly seen in women and girls with autism. Parents are not always experts in autism and will not know what relevant information to present during a diagnostic assessment. It is the clinician's role to prompt parents' recall in specific areas. Many of the questions asked in the Attwood screening test are not those commonly associated with male autism and are therefore not elements that a parent would necessarily think worthy of mentioning.

Gould and Ashton-Smith (2011) also outline a number of key differences in autistic features between girls and boys and recommend a broader view of the diagnostic classification to be taken by clinicians. Items such as increased interest in reading fiction and immersing themselves in fantasy worlds (with set rules that can be followed) are mentioned as needing special consideration. It could be said that no clinician should diagnose (or rule out diagnosis of) autism in females without reference to sex-specific diagnostic materials such as these. It is to be hoped that, in the future, formalised diagnostic tools will become widespread, but in the meantime clinicians must make informed judgements and adjustments to existing tools where necessary. An inexperienced clinician's 'tick box' approach to the autism diagnostic criteria may be very harmful to individuals with a different behavioural profile. An extensive knowledge of autism and face-to-face experience of a significant number of women with autism are necessary. Reading autobiographies, blogs, watching YouTube videos made by women with autism, and spending a day or two at a special school or women's support group, will all help to build the real-life knowledge essential to be a competent clinician.

> The neurobehavioural team [Asperger Syndrome diagnostic service] only takes referrals from consultant psychiatrists in the mental health team, and the mental health team didn't understand autism so wouldn't refer me as they thought that autism was only so-called 'classic' autism and didn't understand that it was a spectrum. (Woman with autism)

Assuming an obvious physical presentation of ASD in a female (or indeed in anyone) may be the first mistake made by an inexperienced clinician. A full picture of childhood behaviours, self-reports and cognitive assessments should form part of the process. As a woman with autism, my own outward observable behaviour in a structured interview situation would not necessarily lead anyone to believe that I have autism, although I can articulate my experience as a person with autism very clearly. There can be a tendency to ignore family and self-reporting, and for the clinician to prioritise what they can 'see'. It is essential to listen to what people say and not make assumptions based on their appearance and presentation. In my professional work, providing non-clinical assessments for individuals who suspect they may have autism, it is extremely rare to find a person who is incorrect about themselves. If an adult has been brought for an assessment by a partner or family member who suspects they have autism, a higher incidence of negative assessment is seen, but when the person investigates and instigates the process themselves, they are usually correct. I don't say this because I am personally seeking to increase the numbers of the autistic population in order to claim world dominance; it is because people do not seek out diagnosis lightly. They have done their research and come to their conclusion solidly before approaching anyone for a diagnosis. As professionals, we must be respectful of the fact that these people are generally not time-wasters. They have more knowledge of themselves – and often their condition – than we do. When they seek diagnosis, frightening comments of professional ignorance are reported: '[UK state diagnostic service] were a disaster – openly admitted they didn't understand autistic girls' (Eaton 2012, p.11), and '[…] the psychologist told me she didn't know girls could get it [autism]' (Eaton 2012, p.11).

> We moved to The Netherlands two years later and she was eventually diagnosed with Asperger Syndrome there at the local Children's Hospital. We thought the Dutch were very liberal and forward thinking but they, to our horror, suggested that A would be better off institutionalised! (Parent of girl with autism)

Increasing the autism education of professionals and clinicians working at all points along the diagnostic and support route has to be the number one priority. In many cases, sadly, this is the stumbling block to accurate diagnosis and appropriate support. A study of mental health professionals in one region of England found that 79 per cent of people rated their own knowledge of autism as 'limited' or 'fair', and 59 per cent said that they had not received any autism training within the past two years. The same study asked service users with autism for their perceptions of Mental Health Services and found that only 17 per cent felt that staff understood their needs relating to having autism and only 23 per cent were satisfied with the mental health support they received (Impact Initiatives *et al.* 2013). Even those who had a positive experience in the end often appeared to have overcome an obstacle course to get there.

> A wonderful psychiatric paediatrician at the local hospital [...] He was the first person who had ever treated us like 'good' parents, who listened to us and to A and was kind, respectful and incredibly helpful. This followed years of horrible professionals giving us misleading diagnoses and making us feel like we were dreadful people. (Parent of girl with autism)

> [The diagnosis] only took a couple of hours looking at school records and history. But took 21 years to get to that stage! We were told at three years old she was retarded! But I knew she was super clever at some things. She was putting sentences together at ten months and hasn't stopped talking since. (Parent of woman with autism)

My experience has been that parents who have had the best outcomes have been those with the confidence and ability to fight for what is their right. Challenging the medical profession is something that many people do not feel comfortable with, but is something that, sadly, is frequently necessary for parents of girls and women with autism.

For older women without parental support, the route to diagnosis is often a solitary one, sometimes met with resistance from professionals. Specialist autism advocacy groups can provide essential support in helping women through the clinical pathway, accompanying them to assessments and supporting them in the collection of relevant lifespan data prior to the diagnostic interview.

> I was told repeatedly by many professionals that I did not NEED a diagnosis but I always felt not fully believed and having to justify myself without one. (Woman with autism)

In order to facilitate accurate diagnosis, it is important for parents and individuals themselves to refer to general autism behavioural characteristic lists and questionnaires focusing on the female behavioural profile (Attwood 2013; Marshall 2014) and take copies of these with them to a diagnostic interview. The Internet is a great resource of behaviour checklists for the autism spectrum condition and there are many books available that outline what to expect. Each item on the characteristics list or questionnaire should be fleshed out with specific examples of how the child/individual would meet each criterion. For an adult, evidence of childhood presentation is also recommended – school reports, conversations with family members and recollections from childhood help to form a life-long picture. In essence, as a person seeking a diagnosis, you should provide as much evidence as possible to support your case to make the clinician's job as easy as possible. This is essential when seeking diagnosis for a female.

As expected, there is a huge range in the ages of individuals and the circumstances in which they or their families first considered that autism might be part of their picture.

> Age four, after reading about how girls manifest their symptoms differently to boys, I just knew. (Parent of girl with autism)

> Random suggestion over lunch with a child psychologist doing a garden tour on the other side of the country. She had just completed a piece of research that matched my daughter's struggles in life after having relationships in adult life that left her vulnerable to violence and financial exploitation. (Parent of woman with autism)

I had always felt 'different' and excluded by others, and wanted to know why. A friend was going for an assessment and I realised I didn't know as much about autism as I thought I did. I read a personal account of having Asperger's by a woman on the Internet and it made me cry with recognition – I knew I had to explore the possibility so that I could at least rule it in or out. (Woman with autism, diagnosed aged 31 years)

My son was diagnosed and as I sat in conferences regarding ASD, I sat there going tick, tick to myself [...] therefore got diagnosis. (Woman with autism, diagnosed aged 37 years)

For some, autism wasn't on their radar, but a definite sense of 'difference' certainly was – and sometimes from a very young age.

When I started school, I noticed everyone else was different to me, but after a while I realised I was the one who was different and not them. (Woman with autism, diagnosed aged 34 years)

We were trying to figure out why all schools kicked her out. Why she had no friends. Why she couldn't keep a job. (Parent of woman with autism)

Both adult women and parents of girls talk about feeling doubt about their conclusions, due to not entirely meeting the traditional (male) profile that proliferates, and not being believed when sharing with others. In the case of some individuals, their lack of general understanding about the spectrum of autism caused them to react negatively when it was suggested as a cause of their child's or their own presentation.

My mother said, 'Do you think she's autistic?' when she was three weeks old. I was furious. She was a very difficult baby for many reasons and it was obvious that she was 'different' from the beginning. I have some severely autistic relatives and I didn't know that there were degrees of autism. I ruled it out because I thought she was much too clever to be 'autistic' [...] It was only when the nursery told me to look up Asperger Syndrome on the Internet that I finally realised what we were dealing with. (Parent of girl with autism)

> I was 26 when I first started to think I could be autistic. I saw something on TV about a girl who had Asperger's [...] I could relate to everything she said. Up until that moment, I thought Asperger's was only found in males. (Woman with autism)

Why diagnose?

For either the parents of a child or the adult themselves, a positive diagnosis of autism is the start of a new journey of understanding, acceptance and adjusted expectations. Formalised processes can begin and appropriate support plans can be implemented. The diagnosis is the key to progress for the individual and their family, and the benefits extend beyond the 'medical' explanation. The importance of a timely diagnosis cannot be over-emphasised.

Psychologically, the family or individual now know what they are facing, so they can move on and deal with it (Eaton 2012). Emotions can be mixed with sadness, guilt and anger, intermittently entwined with relief, acceptance and hope. The reported additional difficulty that females have in obtaining the appropriate diagnosis can make these feelings especially intense. The need to be heard and taken seriously is something shared by many parents of children and adult women on the autism spectrum. The successful diagnosis is evidence that this has happened. The 'vindication' that adult women describe attests to the intensity of this emotion and the importance of diagnosis.

> I hope that armed with this self-knowledge and awareness, the second half of my life will be more productive, fruitful and honest than the first, and that I will no longer feel worthless, stupid and useless and a failure in life. In addition, I wanted to be able to guide my children through their lives in a way that was not available to me. [...] I have begun a journey of self-acceptance and discovery. I am learning who I am and peeling away years of armour and masks to reveal the true essence of the person underneath. I try to be more assertive when negotiating for the small things that make navigating this life easier, and am less apologetic for my quirkiness

and differences that people find so unusual. (Woman with autism, diagnosed aged 41 years)

Child diagnosis

There is an almost universal belief that early diagnosis is a good thing, and certainly that seems to be the case in this day and age where understanding is increasing and appropriate support is possible. However, I have discussed this with some late-diagnosed autistic women friends and colleagues and for us the benefits of early diagnosis are not so clear. Individually, we had all come to the same conclusion that early diagnosis would have meant well-meaning limitations being placed on us by ourselves and those around us – families and teachers – seeking to protect us from undue stress. All of us have significant mental health issues (predominantly anxiety disorders) from pushing ourselves in a world that gave us no concessions, but each of us feels that we have achieved more because of this. In our cases, we feel the label would not have aided our independence.

> There is one disadvantage [to diagnosis] and that is I used to try to convince myself that I was just like everyone else but now I automatically think others will realise I'm different so it puts me off joining up to things which are not autism related. Possibly before I would have been more likely to join. (Woman with autism, diagnosed aged 46 years)

This is our experience, coming from a place where no-one knew or understood. Our bloody-minded determination to fit in at any cost, paid off in terms of our independence, but sometimes at the price of our mental and physical health. Fortunately, girls and young women today have awareness on their side and for them early diagnosis is a positive outcome that may protect them from some of the ancillary mental health issues experienced by older women. The support is there for them. Many of the young women I meet in colleges around the country, where I work, are comfortable with their autism; it's no big deal – they've had it forever. They don't want to talk about it; they just get on with it. It's a totally different experience to the late-diagnosed adult women coming to the realisation for the first time: we want to talk about it, dissect it, analyse it.

Families see one of the major benefits of a child receiving a diagnosis is that it formalises and kick-starts a support process. Families also mention reflecting on their parenting methods and understanding the need to modify these in light of the confirmation of autism. For the families who participated in my research, the diagnosis brought a new and positive sense of direction to their attitude towards their children's care.

> We have stopped trying to use conventional behaviour techniques and adapted them to work [now we understand] why they weren't working in the first place. Mostly, it meant, as parents, we could stop beating ourselves with the 'bad parenting' stick that many people (professional and otherwise) are eager to wield when behaviour is atypical (at best) and dangerous (at worst). (Parent of girl with autism)

> The difference was probably greatest for the family in a psychological sense. We had all been kidding ourselves that she was probably just a bit neurotic and intelligent. When she scored so highly on the ADOS [autism diagnostic tool] it came as a bit of a shock to realise that she was actually quite severely affected in many ways. It has helped us understand and empathise with her better. And it has shut up other members of the family who were convinced she was just 'difficult'! (Parent of girl with autism)

Adult diagnosis

Benefits for adult-diagnosed individuals with autism include being able to access practical support and being taken more seriously by service providers. For many, two of the best things about receiving a diagnosis are the self-knowledge and sense of relief, which can improve self-esteem and confidence, that come from knowing that there was a reason for why they felt so different and for all the challenges they had faced. This is discussed in more detail in Chapter 7.

> It allowed for suitable housing to be gained, benefits to be granted, and a level of explanation I could offer the banks etc. for the out-of-control finances and other severe problems our daughter had at the time. The full weight of the situation began to shift [from being] purely [on] my shoulders, as the mum, to a shared level with others. We were granted 10½ hours a week support – life changing for me! (Parent of woman with autism, diagnosed aged 24 years)

What some people find frustrating, however, is that frequently specialist knowledge stops at the point of diagnosis (Eaton 2012), leaving individuals and families without significant follow-up support or expertise from then onwards.

Post-diagnostic disclosure

Disclosure specifically related to employment is discussed in Chapter 14.

Once the diagnosis of autism has been confirmed, the process of deciding who and how to tell other people begins. Some find that becoming an advocate for autism is a role that they feel comfortable with, celebrating their own or their child's unique self and sharing their knowledge to increase understanding in others. Liane Holliday Willey is an advocate of full disclosure and writes a chapter on it in her book *Pretending to be Normal* (2014), which beautifully portrays the mind of a woman with autism – a must-read for all clinicians and practitioners. For parents, this may mean that they can gain some tolerance for their child's behaviour when things get difficult.

> When we are out and about, my husband and I will explain to people she makes a bee-line for before they have a chance to make judgements (e.g., in restaurants, she will go over and talk to people at their tables and doesn't read the social cues for when they've had enough) and usually this makes people really tolerant and, as she is very endearing, they usually have a lovely interaction. (Parent of girl with autism)

Surprise and disbelief at the diagnosis cropped up frequently for the participants in this book as reactions to their disclosure. This was either because they were girls, or because they 'looked too normal'.

> One person told me, 'I thought that autistic people were retarded and couldn't speak'. (Woman with autism, diagnosed aged 36 years)

> The other friend began treating me like a person with a very low I.Q., doing up my coat if it was cold out, answering for me if I was asked a question, making decisions on my behalf, repeatedly asking me if I was okay etc. It made me feel uncomfortable and slightly ridiculous. (Woman with autism, diagnosed aged 33 years)

> I told people I suspected it was ASD and I got lots of raised eyebrows and 'she's not because she gives eye contact/her language is great/she doesn't flap or rock etc.' but once we had the diagnosis, people were more willing to listen to how girls present very differently. (Parent of girl with autism)

When I received my own diagnosis, the person who carried it out advised me not to be open about it. He said that I was 'not a good advert for autism' and that no-one would believe me because I am too (apparently) capable. He was right about that and gave me this advice with good intent considering his experience of autism and the understanding of women with autism at the time (2010). For three years I told no-one but my immediate family. Even my autistic partner struggled to believe it, as 'my' autism looked quite different to 'his' autism. Even now, my greatest fear, source of indignation and sadness is the disbelief of others. I have not worked out how to respond politely to someone I met only a few minutes ago who tells me, with apparent great authority, that I do not have autism, when every part of my inner being wants to say, 'And how the **** do you know?' and to cry. The experience of being disbelieved about something that feels so hugely fought for is nothing short of devastating. The perception that if the presentation isn't immediately visible then the autism isn't something requiring accommodation is a common, and in my case incorrect, one.

Chapter 3

Infancy and Childhood

By the time I was three years old, my parents knew I was not an average child.

LIANE HOLLIDAY WILLEY (2014, P.18)

Parents whose daughters receive a diagnosis of autism later in life often say that they 'just knew' something was different about their child when she was a baby, or certainly often from a very early age – well before any current formal indicators of diagnosis could possibly be used. If the child has a language or developmental delay, it is more likely that the diagnosis of autism will occur sooner rather than later. The child will alert professional attention due to their lack of reaching early childhood milestones, rather than necessarily any specific autistic behaviour. The autism diagnosis may come at the same time – sometimes as young as two years of age, but often the conclusive diagnosis of an Autism Spectrum Disorder (ASD) is reserved until an older age to ensure that the assessment is correct and consistent over time and natural development. For families with no knowledge or understanding of autism, this can be a huge shock and feel like the end of the world at first.

> We had our suspicions very early on, when A was a young baby, that something was amiss. She didn't smile until much later than her peers, could not instinctively play with peers, [was] very socially awkward, [and had] poor gross and fine motor control etc. But she was very bright verbally and taught herself to read when she was about three. We knew nothing about autism then and it seemed like a horrific condition. A teacher suggested it when A was about six

and we threw up our hands in horror. (Parent of girl with autism, diagnosed aged 6 years)

For children who do not have any learning disability or language delay, a diagnosis of autism would not necessarily be an obvious conclusion under three or four years of age and therefore it is to be expected that diagnosis for these children would come later. This seems to be particularly the case with girls. One study found the average age of diagnosis in girls to be eight years of age (Eaton 2012). Giarelli *et al.* (2010) found that boys were more likely to be given an ASD diagnosis earlier than girls, despite both sexes being identified as having similar language and developmental delays at approximately the same age. The girls were initially given a diagnosis of another condition, meaning that the commencement of appropriate support was delayed. In my participant sample, the earliest diagnosis was at four years of age for a girl with a learning disability, while others without a learning disability were slightly older. It is encouraging to learn that some clinicians are identifying ASD so early in these girls and clearly have a good understanding of how to interpret the diagnostic criteria for the female population.

For the parents of these children there is often not anything 'wrong' with their child that they can define or that requires medical assistance, but more a nagging sense of something being different that they can't quite put their finger on. It might be that play is different, or that the child appears unusually absorbed and in a world of their own (Riley-Hall 2012). This is particularly the case for parents of girls with autism as their behaviour may just be attributed by others as 'shy' (Kreiser and White 2014) in a way that often isn't the case with boys. In my experience, these parents are frequently correct in their intuition, but can often be assumed to be over-anxious or imagining things. Obviously, it is not currently appropriate to make a very early autism diagnosis in all cases, but it may be necessary to note the observations of parents voicing concerns of this nature as at some point in the future this could potentially provide valuable supporting evidence for an autism diagnosis. One girl even had the insight to diagnose herself!

By age eight she was questioning if she was on the autistic spectrum herself. We had already been asking (professionals) and had been fobbed off with the fact she was a girl!! Her brother started going through the diagnostic process when she was eight and he was six. By the time she was nine he had been diagnosed with AS [Asperger Syndrome] and she was convinced she was AS too […] (took another 12 years!). (Parent of girl with autism)

Early childhood indicators

When considering typical expected behaviours of a child with autism, parents of girls and women with autism give us an insight into their world in these early years. Some of these behaviours are not gender-specific and will also be seen in boys, particularly at this early stage, but expectations of how girls 'should' be may impact on how these pre-diagnosis age behaviours are interpreted. It is important that autism remains on the radar when considering the causes of certain behaviours in these girls. We should remember that mental health or more general global delay-type diagnoses are known to be more readily given to females when autism may have been more appropriate (see Chapter 1). Parents' observations about their children's behaviours are frequently made with hindsight; they may have caused concern at the time, but parents often fear being told they are paranoid or over-anxious and keep these niggles to themselves. On reflection, the parents questioned had all noticed early atypical behaviour in their infants and toddlers, which later contributed to the picture they now know to be autism.

Typical very early indicators and parental anecdotal reports relate to characteristics and behaviours that include the following:

- The parent feels a sense of detachment from the baby or young child – often this cannot be further articulated by the parent; it is just a feeling of the baby or child 'being in their own world'.

- Atypical eye contact (either unusually limited or staring).

- A lack of attention paid specifically to people and faces – interest in people is not prioritised over objects.

- Limited interest and/or response to people stimuli (smiling, voices, peek-a-boo games).

- Limited reciprocal social facial expressions and social cues (smiling, pointing).

- Limited seeking out of people and responses from people.

- Very placid, silent and peaceful babies – 'It was spooky, was almost as though she was a ghost just lying there silently without moving.' (Parent of girl with autism)

OR

- Very anxious, distressed and clingy babies – 'Intense emotions, especially distress, and an inability to be comforted by affection.' (Attwood 2012)

- Sensory preferences and intolerances:

    ◦ small temperature tolerance range, which can result in febrile convulsions

    ◦ clothing – texture and touch

    ◦ physical touch – distressed by being cuddled

    ◦ specific strong food preferences and dislikes

    ◦ food and other intolerances and allergies.

Professor Tony Attwood has developed a *Girls' Questionnaire for Autism Spectrum Conditions* (Attwood 2013) for use by clinicians with parents of girls seeking diagnosis, to highlight female-specific characteristics and ensure that a full and accurate profile is provided. This tool is not a diagnostic test for autism in its own right but rather a supplementary information source asking the right questions to get the right information. The questions include items such as toy preference, imaginary friends/animals, adopting personas in different situations and responses to social errors. All of the items on Attwood's screening questionnaire were evidenced in the girls and women questioned for this book and are aspects of autism not usually considered indicative in traditional diagnostic measures. Tania Marshall, a specialist female autism practitioner, has also developed a profile of female traits for both girls and adult women which reflect a broader range than those typically measured diagnostically (Marshall 2013) and also mirrors those discussed here.

As we have learned, girls with an ASD can often do a great job of rote learning and mimicking (typically) intuitive communication cues in order to pull off an effective social performance. However, at a young age, it is unlikely that this learning will be fully embedded and so any difference in social engagement should be evident. It may not be until the child joins a nursery or playgroup that the parent realises that their 'quirky' child is really quite different from her peers. Preferences and behaviour, which in isolation at home are easily managed, may not be so easily accepted in a room full of 20 toddlers. It also may not be until the start of group interaction in formal play settings that the child begins to struggle with the more frequent and numerous social interactions and requirements. Therefore, a child who displayed few difficulties at home may suddenly appear much more affected by potential autism due to the change in her environment and the new expectations placed on her – and this may be particularly the case for girls who may be encouraged towards pretend, group and imaginative play in these settings.

Participants in the research for this book were asked for examples of early atypical behaviours that reflect behaviours associated with the autism diagnostic criteria, along with those identified as being potentially more indicative of female autism. The list of topics featured here is not exhaustive and is not a comprehensive list of diagnostic characteristics. They are topics that came up most frequently in my research as being particularly pertinent for these girls and women.

Non-verbal communication

Difficulties with the expression and reading of non-verbal signals, such as eye contact, facial expressions, tone of voice and body language, are presumed to be the more obvious and visible characteristics of autism. It must be remembered that these are reciprocal skills in typically developing children, which result in not only the ability to 'read' other people, but also to present the appropriate non-verbal signals to enable other people to 'read' them. The child with autism may not only fail to pick up on cues from others and respond to those, but also to make the necessary facial expressions to transmit their own messages outwards to be received by others. Thus, a child who makes few facial expressions, or ones that appear slightly out of context in the situation, is certainly a candidate for consideration of autism in the same way as a child who does not actively respond to cues.

> On holiday aged eight, a kindly hotel owner observed that I never smiled and asked why I always looked so worried. I panicked as I didn't know what to answer, so I came out with the first thing that seemed reasonable to be worried about which was 'the ozone layer'. I must have heard about this on the news. (Woman with autism)

Eye contact was mentioned by parents of girls with autism as being noticeably different in infancy in their daughters. This is something that is typically observed in babies within the first few weeks of life (assuming there are no physical visual problems). Eye contact differences in individuals with autism can range from little or no eye contact through to staring. The difference for a person with autism is in the intuitive understanding of eye contact as a means of reciprocal communication (and therefore not discerning any function in looking at someone's eyes), a difficulty in attending to more than one sensory input at once, or simply an intense discomfort at the intensity of looking into another person's eyes. As an adult, a person with autism may observe that eye contact is a social norm and teach themselves to replicate this (with varying levels of success), while a small child is behaving in their natural state, rather than one with learned modifications.

> While breastfeeding she would pull away if I gazed at her. Whilst in her door-bouncer she would turn around to face the opposite direction if I tried to engage with her. (Parent of girl with autism)

> I have quite a number of memories that date back to two years of age and onward. Most of my memories of people during my toddler

years are of parts of their bodies and not their faces or eyes (e.g. feet, hands, hair). (Woman with autism)

It is important to note that in autism, a lack of eye contact does not equate to someone not understanding or listening. This may give rise to a child being described as a 'daydreamer' or 'in her own little world' when in fact she may be entirely present but not making the socially required non-verbal signals to indicate that she is. It may be that other senses can be utilised more effectively if a person doesn't have to look at the unfathomable movements of a face at the same time.

> I had a reputation in my family as being someone who did not listen to people. Part of that may have been due to the fact that I often did not look directly at them or did not appear to be attending to them when they spoke to me. They would often say: 'Listen! Use your ears… Look at me when I am speaking to you… Pay attention!' (Woman with autism)

Some parents observed differences in other non-verbal communication skills that one would usually expect from even a young child, such as pointing and the showing of items. Robyn Steward (Jansen and Rombout 2014) says that her mother knew she was autistic when she was only a few months old because she didn't cuddle up to her, make eye contact or point at things. Her mother began to sing to her and that's how they connected with each other. Once the diagnosis is made, it may be easier to look back and realise what was happening, although at the time with no reference point it would be difficult to pinpoint the root of specific behaviour, such as asking for reassurance to an unusual degree. This could easily be misconstrued as stemming from anxiety, rather than an inability to receive the required data from a face, for example. For clinicians and other professionals, it is important to consider these individual clues through the lens of autism to ascertain their true origin.

> She misses many non-verbal cues and especially struggles with facial expressions and tone of voice and will regularly ask if someone is cross/happy with her as she isn't sure. (Parent of girl with autism)

I didn't know pointing meant I had to look unless I was explicitly told and I often couldn't tell what the other person was pointing at. I found it pretty useless myself as a communication tool so didn't really use it. (Woman with autism)

There will usually have been some kind of non-verbal or subtle sign that other children do not want her to play, [but] she misses it and the situation escalates. (Parent of girl with autism)

Speech, verbal communication and language comprehension

Language has always been part of the diagnostic criteria for ASDs, but has been dropped in the new DSM-5 criteria as a distinct measure. Individuals with autism present a varied profile across language ability, both in speech and language comprehension. Some individuals are entirely non-verbal throughout their lives, yet may have good intellect and sophisticated understanding. The majority of those questioned for this book had early speech, advanced vocabulary and sometimes 'incessant chatter'. This was the case even when the general learning profile of the child was delayed or weak in other areas. Speech and language were precocious in many of these girls and something that those around them especially noticed. I was one of these children; my mother reported that I spoke full sentences by the time I was nine months old. It is likely that due to the weight given to verbal ability and speech, as indications of both intelligence and social skill, the eloquence of these girls may have distracted parents and clinicians from considering autism as a potential diagnosis.

Aged three, when she had something in her eye, she said, 'I have an obstruction in my pupil'. (Parent of girl with autism)

This may have caused parents and professionals to overlook potential social difficulties, because speech was profuse and advanced in amount and vocabulary, even though it was not necessarily so adept in pragmatics (Attwood 2012). In contrast, these girls were also seen to have social difficulties in understanding social cues and reciprocal relationship development, despite their verbosity and apparent sociability.

> I could speak eloquently by age two. My mother often describes it like I 'swallowed a dictionary' [...] My comprehension of language was always very high though I would use words hollowly; [I knew] the context but not the exact meaning. (Woman with autism)

It is important that speech is not seen as the fundamental measure of intelligence or social skills, as it can be deceptive and misleading for both verbal and non-verbal individuals across the autism spectrum. It is necessary to look beneath the vocabulary and analyse the quality and nature of the communication and relationship dynamics. The words may be scripts learned from a favourite TV show, or overheard on a bus; the meaning might not be understood to the level that the eloquent and precise speech might suggest.

> I spoke on time, but used a lot of echolalic speech (e.g., if I hurt myself, I'd say 'Does it hurt?' rather than: 'I am hurt'). I also used quite pedantic speech with long words and spoke in very formal language. (Woman with autism)

> She has difficulty with idiom, sarcasm, tone of voice, multiple and complex instructions. This becomes increasingly evident as her peers begin to understand these language usages. It was less obvious when she was younger as very few of the children had these skills. (Parent of girl with autism)

Individuals with autism are often described as 'literal', but this does not always fully encompass what this means in reality. One such resulting behaviour can be a wonderful and brutal bluntness and honesty that often accompanies autism at all ages. Many typical children are known to speak their mind and say inappropriate things, but those children will undoubtedly learn from their mistakes and quickly learn the skills of verbal and non-verbal subtlety, which, along with empathy, allow for more gentle interactions. This behaviour can be particularly poorly tolerated in girls, who are expected to be tactful.

> 'Fat grandmothers don't ride bikes.'
> [...] 'Liane, let your grandmother ride your new bike.'

'No. She is too fat and she will break it.' [...]

And off I rode, on my bike, no fat grandmas with me. (Holliday Willey 2001, p.39)

The resulting reprimand for this type of truthfulness is deeply puzzling for the girl with autism who has yet to learn that sometimes honesty is not the best policy.

> I remember being aware when I was about five that older kids did their 'tables', as in times tables. I imagined this involved stacking tables on top of each other and was gutted to find out it didn't. (Woman with autism)

Individuals with autism can be literal, both in their own speech and in interpreting that of others, in ways that a non-autistic person couldn't possibly predict or appreciate. This difficulty in seeing beyond the actual (literal) meaning of what has been said is a constant cause of anxiety for many on the autism spectrum because it generally involves other people (social interaction) and a potential for failure, confusion or something unexpected happening, all of which are stressful and to be avoided. The examples provided by my women respondents were both brilliant and painful, and beautifully illustrate what a baffling and distressing world they had to endure as small children. I could have presented an entire chapter on these head-scratching encounters.

> When I was about seven I asked my mum how old she was and she told me she was 21 (she was in fact about 50!), but I believed her; and when I told my teacher this and my teacher insisted that she couldn't be 21, I felt betrayed, I had no idea why my mother would lie about such a thing. (Woman with autism)

> I was being presented with a perfect attendance award at a school ceremony and I did not respond several times when my name was called. When my mother asked me why I did not respond when my name was called, I told her that I wasn't sure if there were other XXs in the audience (i.e. others having the same first and last name) and I wasn't sure it was me they were talking about. At that time, I did not

know that a person's first name/last name combination was unique to each single person in most instances. (Woman with autism)

My mum organised a costume party. I remember that during the party all I wanted to do was to change in and out of costumes, until I had found the right one. The other girls wanted to play, and they kept telling me they were bored. I did not realise that the reason for a costume party was to play as usual only dressed up. I thought costume parties were to play at changing costumes. (Woman with autism)

Dealing with unpredictability

The inheritability of autism can be a blessing for some girls growing up with autism in families where similar characteristics may be inherent in parents:

We had a set routine and saw few new people. We didn't go on holidays or visit new places and did not have birthday parties. I did not have to cope with much change [...] I think my parents were both on the spectrum and liked what was familiar. (Woman with autism)

The fight or flight response to unexpected situations and occurrences is well documented in autism and reported by parents describing their girls' behaviour. Parents can find themselves needing to be alert to potential triggers in order to maintain the safety of their children. Alternatively, parents struggle with a child whose response to an unpredictable world is to avoid it at all costs and remain alone at home. Parents can feel that their daughter 'should' be sociable, and they experience extreme guilt and sadness at her perceived isolation, whereas the child herself feels quite happy, calm and safe at home engaged in her own interests.

She would prefer to stay at home and never go out, so life is stressful for all of us trying to persuade her to lead a normal life. (Parent of girl with autism)

We are able to change routines if we do it slowly and give her a good explanation and a long enough presentation period (this is tricky as it is dependent on the situation – if we introduce a change or proposed trip too early, then she has increased anxiety and obsessive questioning!). (Parent of girl with autism)

Activity choice

Choice of play can be one of the earliest indicators of autism (Riley-Hall 2012). Interestingly, one of the findings from research into sex differences in children with autism was that girls with autism do not have the same stereotypical, rigid interests as boys (Carter *et al.* 2007). My research certainly found that repetitive and restricted behaviours were completely the norm for the girls studied but that topic type differed. A small number of activities came up time and time again as being favourites for repetition: watching the same TV/video/DVD programme (e.g., *Mary Poppins*, *Postman Pat*, *Peppa Pig*), reading the same book (e.g., an Enid Blyton book, *Jane Eyre*), listening to the same song/tape. The scripts and lyrics of their favourite shows, books and songs were all known verbatim by the children.

> As an eight-year-old girl, I knew the entire songs and dialogue to the films: *Sound of Music*, *Chitty Chitty Bang Bang*, *Annie* and *Mary Poppins*. (Woman with autism)

Collecting and sorting specific objects were also mentioned. I recall spending many hours attempting to devise an efficient means of systemising my extensive collection of Lego®, but was conflicted about the criteria that should be applied – size of block, colour or function – and never succeeded in finding a system that satisfied me. It still disturbs me when contemplating my grandchildren's Lego.

Although this is still the same core behaviour associated with autism, I think that there is a qualitative difference between male 'lining up' behaviour and female behaviour. The girls' activities generally involve people, rather than objects (aside from an almost universal love of Lego). These people may be fictional characters, or only their voices are heard (in the case of music), but the girls' interest in them is all people-based, rather than purely object-based (dinosaurs, buses etc.). The girls' behaviour also all involves words and communication on some level.

Given the early and advanced speech mentioned by many interviewed, there does appear to be – in my sample at least – some desire for communication, language or words by these girls at an early age, even if the purpose and intuitive understanding of the social rules are not necessarily present. Surely it is no coincidence that, despite reported numbers of women with autism being significantly lower than those of men, many of the most established and prolific authors in autism – particularly those telling their own story – are women. Perhaps women with autism have an innate drive to communicate.

> (She) would act out scenarios she had witnessed (real or books or films). The same scenes would be played over and over again [...] She would always include the 'he said' or 'she said' after dialogue – as if she was reading from a book. (Parent of woman with autism)

Intense interests

> I developed an interest in *Coronation Street*. Now, it is quite typical to enjoy soap operas, and I knew that it was perfectly okay for me to ask my classmates if they had watched the previous evening's episode. I knew it wasn't perfectly okay for me to tell them how many bricks the Rovers Return was made out of or the exact dates each character had made their first appearance, how I was making a scale model of the set. (Mason, in Hurley 2014, p.14)

Enjoying an intense interest in one or more subjects is a core element in the profile of autism, but differences in the specifics of this profile are noted between boys and girls (Attwood 2012). Boys' interests tend to be object-based – trains, dinosaurs, space – while girls' interests tend to be people- or animal-based – soap operas, fictional characters, animals and celebrities. This qualitative difference can explain why girls' behaviour may not be noted as being unusual, due to the 'typical girl' nature of their interests (Simone 2010; Wagner 2006). Whereas a boy who quotes endless facts about ancient history, rather than playing football with his peers, may be flagged as atypical, a girl who obsesses about a pop star would not necessarily be seen in the same way. The difference between the interests of a girl with autism and a typical child is the narrowness of the topic and the intensity of the interest. These girls with ASD have single-track focus; they do not think or speak of anything other than their passion for an extended period. They may have extensive knowledge of their subject but have more of a factual interest than a desire to live it out. A child who speaks of nothing but horses may not actually want a horse, but just enjoys the facts about horses. I believe that the interest provides the same outcomes for both girls and boys on the autism spectrum; once immersed in your subject of interest, there is a predictability and escape from the chaotic real world. Knowing everything about a subject makes it known and provides a sanctuary from the anxiety and stress of a feeling of not knowing what's going to happen most of the time.

Animals in general are a popular interest as they are far easier to deal with than people for many females with autism: their intentions are clear (no hidden agendas), their non-verbal language is minimal (cats don't pull too many facial expressions), their needs are easily identified and their attachment and affection are unconditional and unchanging. Some girls identify so strongly with animals that they imagine or wish themselves to be one (Attwood 2007).

> I was a pony before I had one. I cantered everywhere, neighed out loud and jumped imaginary obstacles. (Woman with autism)

I would suggest that animals are more of a favourite interest for girls than for boys with autism. As previously mentioned, there does seem to be a desire for many of these girls to connect in some way with living beings (people, animals, insects) rather than just with inanimate objects, as the boys tend to do. The nature of this connection, however, may be significantly different than that experienced by typical children.

Typical interests of a girl on the autism spectrum

These interests include the following:

- animals – cats, horses

- nature

- soft toys

- characters from books

- collecting

- TV programmes

- TV/movie actors

- historical characters.

I collected lots of items, from key rings to daddy longlegs (insect) […] I had an old jar that I filled to bursting with these insects; really awful when I think back to these creatures suffering. I loved to look at them in the jar; I was fascinated with them moving about crammed together. (Woman with autism)

She gets fixated with certain people who she admires. These can be real (e.g., an older girl at school), historical (e.g., Princess Vicky, daughter of Queen Victoria), or imagined (e.g., a character from a book or film). (Parent of girl with autism)

After reading *The Hobbit* and *Lord of the Rings*, she learned the two languages – Quenya and Elvish – and spent hours writing them. (Parent of girl with autism)

Toy choice

In those asked, toy preference in girls was overwhelmingly driven towards toys designed for 'doing', rather than imagining or pretending. Knickmeyer *et al.* (2008) found that girls with autism did not show a preference for female-typical items when engaged in play that did not involve pretence. Cars, Lego®, construction, Pokémon™, robots and monsters all featured. For me in the 1970s it was Airfix® models along with the cars and Lego®. Even for girls who loved having soft, cuddly toys and dolls, the play was more in organising, collecting and sorting rather than interactive and imaginative play with these items.

> I must have been around two years old when my grandmother gave me a doll. I remember how much I disliked it. I put it in the bin. (Woman with autism)

The girl with ASD may have more dolls than her peers, but these may be arranged in a specific order and not used for shared imaginative play (Attwood *et al.* 2006). For those girls who did play out scenarios with teddies and dolls, it is generally anecdotally reported by parents and individuals to often be verbatim scripts of earlier events or replications of parental behaviours. One child would re-enact her school day word for word with her toys at home (this was verified by the parent asking the teacher about the day). On first appearance, these activities can look very typical and imaginative, but this may not always be the true picture. A child who talks to herself out loud and puts on different voices may not be creating imaginary characters and complex worlds, but may be repeating TV shows, conversations and events that she has actually experienced. It is important that accurate and detailed information about the content of the play is gathered, as taking the observation at face value may be misleading.

> When she does play with girls' toys, she has very prescriptive play – undresses them all and puts them all to bed – with no story or interaction between dolls. (Parent of girl with autism)

> Gave my soft toys idiosyncratic or functional names – Best Ted, Fat Ted ('Fat' used in a descriptive rather than a derogatory sense). (Woman with autism)

Some girls in my sample didn't play with any toys at all, preferring to be outside, active and enjoying nature. Tony Attwood includes an interest in nature in his *Girls' Screening Questionnaire* (Attwood 2013).

> I did not play with the typical toys; I preferred to be outside running free. (Woman with autism)

Other commonly reported activities included colouring, collecting items and reading. Many girls with ASD are self-taught readers (Simone 2010), learning quickly and voraciously devouring any book they can find, whether information-based or fiction. As Rudy Simone says: 'Information replaces confusion' (Simone 2010, p.23). Not only does reading offer a solo escape from a chaotic world, it also provides knowledge and data that may help the girl to manage that world once she has to return to it. Shared pretend play didn't appeal to many of the girls in my survey; they preferred to be 'doing' rather than 'being', unless, that is, they were immersed in a solo fantasy world of their own creation; more about that in a moment.

Encouraging interests and desire for knowledge is a good way to support and motivate a girl with ASD. Parents and professionals may be concerned about her isolation and lack of social interaction, but it may be that school or family life overwhelms her far more quickly than it does other children, and allowances need to be made for her to be alone in order to replenish her capacity. If this is not appreciated, eventual shutdown, meltdown and/or increased anxiety will be the almost inevitable result.

> She loves books and plays with them as well as reading them – almost like they have their own personalities. (Parent of girl with autism)

Play was almost exclusively solo for the girls in my sample under the age of around six years, although some girls did seek out the company of others, but found that it only took a very short time for them to either offend the other children or become upset with the notion of shared play. The girl appears to take either a domineering role, in which all activities have to be on her terms, or a more passive role where she is 'mothered' by more socially able girls. These findings back up another study (Knickmeyer *et al.* 2008) that found that girls did not show a preference for 'female-typical' items in non-pretence play, whereas boys with autism did show a preference for 'male-typical' items. In pretend play, girls with autism show a preference for same sex-typical toys (as do boys with autism). One suggestion is that girls with autism are more likely to have learned how to do pretend play from their parents, as this is often more encouraged in girls than in boys. Girls, as we have heard, also appear to be motivated to learn how to fit in and behave as expected of a typical girl and this may demonstrate a high capability for imitation.

For the few girls who did play with dolls and more traditional female toys, in most cases parents and individuals reported that this appeared to be more from an awareness of what was acceptable and required by other girls in order to be considered for social interaction and friendship.

> A likes pink and princesses. I think this is because the other girls like them – she doesn't actually play with her princess dolls unless her friends are playing with them. She much prefers to be outside collecting flowers and insects. (Parent of girl with autism)

Fantasy worlds

One of the common anecdotally reported differences between the male and female presentation of autism concerns the concept of imaginative play, as discussed above. Traditionally, children with autism are considered to not engage in imaginary play due to a limited ability to generate fictional worlds and ideas. The observation of play is normally part of the diagnostic assessment, and the classic lining up of cars that many people associate with autism is thought to be a clear indicator of differences or limits in the typically expected imagination. In girls, however, something different is sometimes seen, which may seem contradictory to the comments presented above that stated that girls were less creative in their games. Individually and privately, girls with autism are known to sometimes inhabit a rich fantasy world full of imaginary friends, animals and creatures (Attwood 2007; Holliday Willey 2014). Having imaginary friends is not particularly unusual for any child, but as Tony Attwood (2007) says, 'the child with Asperger's syndrome [sic] may *only* have friends who are imaginary, and the intensity and duration of the imaginary interactions can be qualitatively unusual' (p.25).

> I much preferred the company of my imaginary friends. Penny and her brother Johnna were my best friends, though no one saw them but me. My mother tells me I used to insist that we set them places at the table, include them on our car trips, and treat them like they were real beings. (Holliday Willey 2014, p.19)

> The biggest universe I ever created originally contained about 100 creatures, but this is now over 1000, as this universe has stuck with me throughout my entire life [...] This fantasy is a place I would often slip into as a child, especially when I wished to avoid other people. I had in excess of 64 imaginary friends and I much preferred playing with these characters than interacting with anyone at all. (Woman with autism)

I believe that this is not a contradiction but represents a difference in what girls with ASD present visibly in terms of play and games (often when others are involved), and what really goes on in their private worlds inside their heads where there are no boundaries, restrictions or social rules. Having no interest in fiction is an indicator on some autism assessment tools that were developed through investigation of the male profile (due to larger numbers of males available for sampling, rather than any deliberate intent to exclude females). However, overwhelmingly what we see in girls is an unusual extreme identification with the characters in fiction books, TV programmes and sometimes people they know and feel an attachment to; the girls actually 'become' the character. This may involve re-enacting scenes from the book, film or show over and over again, mimicry and getting lost in the fantasy to the point of having difficulty in separating it from real life. As mentioned previously, we also see girls who identify far more closely with animals than humans and believe and behave as though they are a cat, for example. One young woman, aged 18, whom I worked with, said that she didn't want to grow up as adulthood seemed too scary, and that if she were a cat, people would take care of her. She would often wear a tail and cat ears.

> She was obsessed with Postman Pat's cat, Jess, and would like to be talked to as a cat and reply in cat language. (Parent of woman with autism)

From a diagnostic perspective, it is possible that this could be viewed as delusion or psychosis, whereas for the girls I spoke to, it was more of an escape to a better place from a real world that was difficult and sometimes unhappy.

> I used to disappear to some local hilly fields and roam around pretending I was Maria, from *The Sound of Music*, singing my head off. Fantasy was my escape. In my pretend world, I was an amazing, talented girl. (Woman with autism)

> I much preferred my imaginary world to reality and would spend as much time as I could (apart from when I was reading) thinking about my fantasy world. I often hated getting out of bed because that was a great place to think about my imaginary friends undisturbed, and having to drag myself away from that and return to reality was horrible and depressing. (Woman with autism)

Sensory tolerance

> My number one preferred activity as a toddler and young child, was rocking including: rocking on my duck, rocking on my rocking horse, rocking on my bed or rocking on the floor. (Woman with autism)

Observable sensory differences can present themselves early on for children on the autism spectrum and these are likely to be made known in no uncertain terms by an infant or small child. Refusal, screaming and general extreme distress when encountering specific objects or sensations may be an indicator of an inability to tolerate something. Equally, for those who discover a sensory experience that soothes and calms, a seeking out and incessant desire for that stimulus might be noted. Some of these behaviours originate from external sensory stimuli such as noise or tactile textures, while others are self-generated and found to be either enjoyable in their own right, or are used as a self-soothing strategy or means of communication in times of stress. W. Lawson (1998) describes a rich world of sounds and sensations and says that she was aware that her peers had not noticed these in the way that she had. Her world was made both stressful and soothed by different sensory experiences.

> I did not understand why I was afraid to touch but now I think it caused lots of sensations that were overwhelming for me. It also called for some form of response, which meant having to make a decision. Decisions were confusing for me and it was easier to play it safe and stay with what was familiar. (Lawson 1998, p.41)

Liane Holliday Willey (2014) describes how many noises and bright lights made her life unbearable and that she found relief underwater in her 'safety zone' (p.28). Most of the women and parents I questioned list a considerable number of sensory preferences notable from infancy. For those writing as late-diagnosed adults, we cannot always know what these behaviours were attributed to (if anything) when these women were children, but the frequency and severity of some of the behaviours make it difficult to believe that they were not noticed at the time.

> We have many photos of her squishing her face into mesh fabrics, rolling naked in fleece materials, drinking mud from a trowel! (Parent of girl with autism)

> She used to like to push her forehead against the drum of the washing machine on full cycle to feel the vibrations and would put paper bags on her head as a toddler and just run until she crashed into things. (Parent of girl with autism)

> She has a stereotypical whole body tic when excited which involves opening and closing her hands while twisting the wrists, curling and flexing her feet and opening her mouth all at the same time. (Parent of girl with autism)

Food

> 'Marmalade and cheese!' my friend exclaimed in horror.

> 'Yes, it's even nicer with banana.' (Lawson 1998, p.6)

As with many aspects of the autism profile, behaviours and preferences around food cover more than one element of the diagnostic criteria. Food can represent sensory tolerances, control, preference for sameness and predictability (and therefore avoidance of new and unknown experiences), as well as a different understanding of the social role of food. Specific criteria and rules regarding colour, texture, type, combinations, proximity of one item to another, times, smells and tastes are a relatively common feature in girls with autism. W. Lawson (1998) talks of her need to 'mix and mash up my food' (p.5) in order to cope with different textures, and also of feeling 'afraid' of trying new foods at school, which resulted in her hardly eating any lunch for six months. At this young age, it may be difficult to distinguish typical child phases and fads from something more complex and indicative of autistic-type behaviours, and as a standalone behaviour, this would not be in any way conclusive. Combined with other indicators, however, the child's behaviour around food can add weight to a potential diagnosis.

> I couldn't tolerate lumpy foods or foods that were undercooked. I also had tomato ketchup with virtually everything in order to mask its taste. I was very sensitive to taste and liked things that were either sweet or very bland. (Woman with autism)

> I like to eat my food on a certain plate specific to each different meal or type of food. If I can't use that plate for some reason, it feels wrong and unsettling. (Woman with autism)

> She began to express preferences for three or four food types around the ages of two to three [...] She would change preferences overnight and want the next three or four food types constantly. She still eats like this now and rotations last about six months. (Parent of girl with autism)

Clothing

Universally, for those responding there was a strong preference for clothing that was comfortable, soft, stretchy, loose and smooth. For many, there was also a distinct dislike of clothes that the child considered to be 'girly' (their word). So, not only is there a sensory preference or dislike regarding certain textures, colours or fabrics, but an active choice around types of clothing (skirts, dresses) typically associated with girls. Kopp and Gillberg (2011) report 'careless with physical appearance' as a feature specific to girls with autism. I would question the use of the word 'careless' in this assessment, which is an external, observational judgement. The individual themselves may have taken great care in avoiding certain clothing or textures – the results may look 'careless' or atypical, but may be anything but. It could be suggested that clothing choice in this form may also illustrate something about gender identity and social conformity at an early age in these girls, a subject that will be discussed in greater detail in Chapter 10. Certainly, these girls and women were not generally likely to suffer discomfort in the name of fashion (which is surely a measure of social awareness).

> I preferred jogging bottoms sweatshirts as they were made of soft, smooth, slightly stretchy fabric. Wool clothes physically hurt me and non-stretchy clothes felt stifling, no matter what their size. (Woman with autism)

> She tends to opt for quite outlandish outfits and isn't bothered by what her friends will think or what is fashionable. (Parent of girl with autism)

> [She] has an intense dislike of clothes [...she] will take them off as soon as she walks through the door and in any household where she knows she can. (Parent of girl with autism)

> I like things to be tight around my waist and not tight around my neck. I hate socks and tend to wear them inside out to get the horrid stitching feeling away from my nails. (Woman with autism)

Toileting and personal hygiene

One of the unexpected outcomes of my questions was the high number of girls who had had difficulties in becoming independent with regard to toileting. Toileting issues are commonly reported in individuals with autism, so this should not come as a surprise: social rules, sensory issues and unpredictability are all involved in toileting and personal hygiene. What was surprising was that the majority of these girls did not have any intellectual disability and some were academically extremely intelligent. It could be expected that a child with limited language and understanding may be confused, frightened and distressed by the experience of going to the toilet, but I would have predicted this to be less so for those with greater intellectual capability. The causes may be varied, but anxiety and Irritable Bowel Syndrome are well documented anecdotally as issues for individuals with autism and it is possible that this could make it harder for a child to keep themselves clean. Obviously, it is important to rule out physical causes for toileting difficulties before making assumptions that they are psychological.

> I didn't use the toilet completely independently until I was around 11 as I needed help to wipe my behind on defecating. I eventually learned to do this myself, but had problems with what I now know to be Irritable Bowel Syndrome my entire life, including childhood. (Woman with autism)

> Late to train, but because of extreme fear of poo not her inability to hold and use the toilet. It took ages for her to wipe herself, through worry of poo; she used baby wipes at first and then moved on to toilet roll. (Parent of girl with autism)

> When I was two or three, I had a special toilet seat and would not go to the toilet unless it was on that special seat. (Woman with autism)

> I wet my bed until I was 15 years old. (Jansen and Rombout 2014, p.99)

Participants cited difficulties with recognising the physical signals that indicated a need to go to the toilet, as well as anxiety around using toilet facilities outside their own homes. An expectation that toilet and hygiene rules and behaviour would be intuitive was reported by some women, who were aware that they had 'got this wrong' because the context of why these things were important (and how to do them properly) was assumed to be understood and therefore not taught.

> I was punished severely for not cleaning myself properly [...] If only they had just shown me how to do it properly. (Woman with autism)

> I didn't really understand the purpose of personal hygiene. When I started boarding, aged eight, some of the other girls noticed I didn't clean my teeth, so I became more self-aware of things like this. I still only clean my teeth when I'm going to see other people or if it's been about three days since I last brushed and they feel dirty. (Woman with autism)

Sleep

Sleep is often a problem for children (and adults) on the autism spectrum, but is also typically varied in all babies and infants. For some, bedtime brings respite from a stressful waking day, while for others it brings a new period of confusion and fear. Febrile convulsions featured in several responses and having a 'fuzzy, buzzy head' (Stewart 2012, p.43) was also mentioned by several girls. Anxiety about being left to fall asleep alone, night-time waking and distress, and needing someone to sleep next to them were also commonly mentioned. Poor sleeping patterns were reported by almost all of the participants, mainly due to the reasons cited above. Sleep difficulties are often reported in children with autism although causes are not conclusive. As well as anxiety, ruminating thoughts and sensory difficulties (temperature, textiles) may contribute. These issues can last a lifetime for some people, causing considerable health and occupational difficulties plus associated anxiety (about not being able to sleep).

> From birth to eight months she cried all day and slept all night. She often slept 14 hours a night, she was so exhausted. (Parent of girl with autism)

She complains that she cannot get to sleep because her 'head is busy and there are spots and lines when I close my eyes'. (Parent of girl with autism)

Have always counted to go to sleep [...] this was a tool I used to stop myself thinking about other things which would depress me. I knew that when I could no longer concentrate on one number coming after the last I was very tired and would soon sleep; however, sometimes I reached over 1000. (Woman with autism)

Gender identity in childhood

Research suggests that girls and women with autism may have a more masculinised or androgynous neurological profile (Baron-Cohen 2002; Bejerot *et al.* 2012). This is discussed in more detail in Chapter 10 on adult gender identity and sexuality, but for many females with autism, evidence of this becomes apparent at a much earlier age. It is important to consider that the outward presentation of clothing or toy choice does not necessarily represent the internal cognitive profile. Some girls with autism wear pink and play with dolls, but their brain and thought processes tend to be more pragmatic, logical and less socially intuitive than a neurotypical female.

Not tomboy. Very girly, but do have logical and pragmatic brain. Not very emotional: like steady even dispositions. Don't like games and drama. Hate pink; prefer blue and red or navy and white. (Woman with autism)

Of those participating, 75 per cent felt that they did not specifically identify with behaviours typically associated with girls, even at a young age. This was reported both by parents of girls and by adult women, but as mentioned above, it tends to be viewed diametrically, as either male or female, when in fact it may be simply a more gender neutral behaviour. The majority of respondents used the word 'tomboy' (this word was deliberately not used in the question and was offered by the participants themselves). For those who didn't have a preference for typically boyish behaviour, they identified with something more androgynous:

> I didn't identify as either a boy or a girl (even though intellectually, I knew I was female). I identified more as an android or alien as I didn't believe I could possibly be a human as I was too different from my peers and could see things and see truths about life that they couldn't. (Woman with autism)

> I hated the colour pink with a passion. I wanted to be a plumber when I grew up. Sadly this was frowned upon. I think I probably would have made a good plumber and earned a good wage. (Woman with autism)

> I don't feel girly but I can do my act, and I would never want to be a princess. I'd rather be a superhero or action man! (Woman with autism)

> I related to boys easier, and I had more fun with them. Sometimes I would wish I was a boy; it all seemed so much easier for them. I never understood girls. (Woman with autism)

I hope that the evidence presented so far broadens thoughts about how the profile of a young girl could provide clear evidence for a diagnosis of an ASD when viewed through the lens of autism, rather than viewed through a lens that believes girls don't have autism.

Chapter 4

Childhood Relationships

[B]eing alone did not really bother me – I was happy with my own company. One thing that did disturb me was how other people seemed to enjoy each other's company and actively sought friendships and relationships.

LAWSON (1998, P.57)

Friends and other people

It is a widely held view that individuals with Autism Spectrum Disorder (ASD) have a different understanding and requirement for social interactions from neurotypical people, and being a 'loner' is often considered part of the autism profile. This is not always the case. For some girls with autism, their proactive sociability can be a clue in itself. It is possible to be *too* sociable (according to expected norms), with too few boundaries and little understanding of the feelings and intentions of others. Females on the autism spectrum include individuals who don't engage at all or who actively avoid interaction, but also those who don't know when not to engage and who reveal differences in knowing what to do, how often and when to stop. The skills involving theory of mind and the development of intuitive empathy are not developed until around four years of age in typically developing children, and so cannot be indicative of potential autism in a child under this age.

She is incredibly sociable and seeks interaction with anyone she meets [...] With adults it can make her vulnerable – she wanted to cuddle the telephone engineer and the dog food delivery man (when she was six or seven) [...] when she 'takes a shine' to someone, she will not be swayed. (Parent of girl with autism)

When I did interact, it was inappropriate. For example, as a young toddler I would sometimes seek out physically stimulating activities or rough play with certain adults, such as rubbing up against them, rocking in their lap, seeking to have my back or my arms scratched or tickled, roughly playing with their hair or their hands, etc. (Woman with autism)

Difficulty understanding the rules and expectations of social situations is a common feature of autism, and one that requires not only verbal and non-verbal interpretation and expression, but also a kind of cultural understanding of what is required and expected in any given, specific setting. Individuals with autism may lack some of these subtle observational abilities and need more direct guidance in order to know how to act. It seems to me that individuals with autism have to learn mechanically (consciously) what others learn intuitively (unconsciously).

I was constantly being trained by my mother on how to read the non-verbal cues of others and how to say the right things at the right time. We often role-played what to do and say in various situations. I was not very good at generalising from one situation to the next. It's almost as if I had to know the specific script for each situation and encounter, no matter how similar the situations might be to a past experience. (Woman with autism)

Again, for girls, the expectation is that they will be naturally good at this extremely subtle, intuitive, nuanced skill that requires adaption from moment to moment. For females with autism this cannot be assumed, and care should be taken not to reprimand a girl more severely than one would a boy with autism behaving in a similar fashion. It is also important to recognise this behaviour in girls for what it is, rather than attribute it to another (perhaps intentional) reason.

For most of the girls and women who participated in my research, there was some desire to interact with people, and often a sense of a conscious awareness of finding it difficult – despite the desire to do it – from a young age. They appeared to process the experience consciously rather than intuitively, observing the situation almost from a distance and working out what to do, but often missing some important element, for example what it is to have a friend and be a friend. This suggests that a huge amount of early awareness and cognitive processing is required. One can imagine that this would be isolating, exhausting and baffling for a young child with autism, and that they might also have a sense that everyone else just seems to 'get it'.

> Playtime was very difficult. I didn't know how other kids just sort of knew what to do and who to play with. So, I just hung out by myself, wandered around the playground, sometimes standing weirdly in a group of kids, not saying much, thinking that was enough to be included and considered a part of whatever game they were playing. Mostly I just watched. (Woman with autism)

> I remember feeling like I should play one-to-one, because no one else played alone, but I didn't know how to make it happen. (Woman with autism)

Certainly, some women were not forthcoming in seeking interaction and actively avoided doing so. Liane Holliday Willey (2014) recalls an overwhelming desire to be away from her peers in her earliest years, much preferring the company of her imaginary friends. In either case, whether silent or actively seeking an audience, most of the girls in my sample were typically not considered as potentially autistic until they had reached adulthood, despite what, with hindsight, can be seen as clear indicators of some difference. On reflection, it is easy to attribute their behaviour to shyness, or even high intelligence in some cases, but when combined with a broad profile and an understanding of autism, indications of their future diagnosis are not difficult to see.

> Other people are just walking noise machines. I didn't wish to be around them and desperately wanted to be alone much of the time. (Woman with autism)

Playtime for A would consist of running up and down the perimeter of the fence, flapping and clapping her hands and having an inner dialogue with herself. (Parent of girl with autism)

Preference for adults

Seeking adult interaction, rather than peer interaction, from a young age appears to be a common feature of many girls on the autism spectrum, with around 60 per cent of those asked saying that adults were their first choice of companion. Mothers and grandparents were favourite companions, with some girls not requiring or seeking anyone in the world other than these people as a playmate.

A just wants to be with me. She tells me this all the time. (Parent of girl with autism)

I rarely sought out people and when I did it was for a specific task or to play a specific game or get help with a piece of work. I didn't ever seek out people just for idle chit chat or to play their games or because I wanted a hug or any other such nonsense. I preferred the company of adults. (Woman with autism)

Adults are less complicated than peers to engage with and their communication is usually clearer. As a child, my preferred choice for my birthday party was an evening of card games with a family that my Mum had known her entire life: two elderly parents and their adult children. I was the only child. I never had any birthday party other than this. And never wanted one. The idea of being the centre of attention in a social gathering of children would have been a horrific thought.

These girls in my survey describe friendships on their terms, sometimes with little perception or regard for the feelings of others, even after theory of mind had kicked in for their peers. These girls were making fewer – or at least more socially clumsy – attempts at connecting with peers from a very young age than would be expected from a typically developing child.

A really wanted to relate to adults or older children. She didn't seem to 'get' how to be with her peers […] She would rather hit someone over the head or cover them in paint, which didn't endear her to either them or their parents. (Parent of girl with autism)

Peer friendships

From the participants' responses, 50 per cent were considered 'shy' as young children, a view that is also found in the literature (Giarelli *et al.* 2010; Riley-Hall 2012). A small number fell into the 'overpowering' category, where the wants of the other children were not taken into consideration; but in general, these girls were quiet – unusually quiet. This quietness does not alert professionals to any potential difficulties – quiet is harmless and isn't causing any trouble. The responses from participants give us an insight into what was really going on behind that quiet exterior.

On my first day of kindergarten, I hid behind my mum's legs and stood with her and the other parents, staring at the kids. I had absolutely no desire to socialise with them or to play. (Woman with autism)

Some of the women questioned had a strong sense of being tolerated by other children, rather than actively liked. The effect of this awareness must have had a considerable impact on self-esteem and well-being.

I made a few friends from my class, all of whom bossed me around and eventually got sick of me. Whenever I didn't have any friends from my class, I'd play with kids from younger classes, but even they would eventually point out that I should play with kids my own age. (Woman with autism)

Around 25 per cent of the women questioned had experienced bullying as children. Bullying among the autistic population is old news and it is rare in my work that I meet a person with ASD who hasn't been bullied at school and beyond. It is possible that for some of these girls, their 'shyness', invisible presentation and quiet demeanour may have protected them from bullying to some degree. Perhaps those girls who were bullied were more obviously different in some way, which made them an easy target. Many of the responses give the impression that the girls were mostly simply left alone, as they were of very little interest to bullies (or anyone else for that matter), but, sadly, that wasn't always the case.

> I was constantly being bullied. A lot of the times even by the people I considered to be my best friends. I was picked last on the team, not invited to parties, called names, and once they even put glue on my chair. (Woman with autism)

That is not to say that all girls with ASD are the passive type. Some girls can be loud, outspoken and come across as aggressive or dictatorial, needing to control any interactions and struggling when games change or things don't go their way. The child can appear serious and intolerant of others whom they perceive are 'doing it wrong'.

> My sister says that when we were kids she was always under the impression that she was annoying me [...] I remember being very authoritarian and wanting to dictate to them [siblings] how to play. (Woman with autism)

For these girls their social difficulties can manifest in a more pro-active, socially clumsy and sometimes overpowering way. Eileen Riley-Hall (2012) suggests that there is less tolerance from teachers for aggression in girls than in boys, and that girls, from an early age, are expected to be more polite and considerate of others' feelings.

> I was something of a tyrant [...] but only to those I viewed as wrongdoers. I had a keen sense of justice even at that age; but to those who ended up on my naughty list, so to speak, I would act almost animalistic towards them and was pulled out of the group for physical aggression. (Woman with autism)

> Sometimes I was a bully, especially when I spent time with younger kids. They would get me to go and hit a child they didn't like and

this would make me popular with them, so I did it. (Woman with autism)

I was quite violent; when I couldn't communicate what was wrong I think I just let my fists do the talking. (Woman with autism)

Girls with ASD may appear to have friends or, more accurately, often just one friend, so the child doesn't appear to be particularly isolated or a 'loner'. For some girls, this one friend can become a life-line and help her to gain access into the social arena. The friend can become a subject of fascination and focus, which can cause enormous distress if and when she decides she wants to play with other children.

From a very young age, I craved exclusivity with a 'best friend'. (Woman with autism)

In other cases, women with ASD say that large groups were the best places for them, as they could hide on the peripheries with little requirement to participate (Attwood 2007).

I did attach to the most 'high status' group of friends at my primary school […] as they served a purpose for me in reducing the bullying I faced […] I wouldn't really call that 'friendship' though, it was more an interaction of convenience. (Woman with autism)

Larger groups meant I could smile, laugh, agree and hide away, camouflaged by the group identity. (Woman with autism)

The girls' friends are sometimes very similar to them – other girls who find the social whirl difficult for various reasons; or they are very different – super-sociable girls who scoop up the stragglers and mother them. All of this leads the casual observer to conclude that all is well in the social world of the girl with ASD.

They (friends) were those that were considered outlandish for various reasons. (Woman with autism)

I describe her [friend] as a 'social crutch'. (Parent of girl with autism)

> Her friends have been foreign children with a different language.
> (Parent of girl with autism)

The other common friends for girls with ASD are boys. We have already seen that the vast majority of girls and women with ASD identify themselves as 'tomboys' and find other girls to be far more complex and nuanced in their social skills than boys. This is particularly the case in the teenage years when friendships change from being interest-based to being more personality-based and the girl with ASD can struggle to keep up with the multiple and involved intricacies of female teenage relationships (more on this in Chapter 5).

> I wanted to play with boys at school. I don't think I understood other girls and did not feel comfortable with them, always whispering and giggling. Girls are not nurturing, they are mostly bitchy and cliquey. (Woman with autism)

> I did not understand the girls' group dynamics. I was always on the periphery and I felt very inadequate. (Woman with autism)

Copying

We have noted that girls with autism learn how to behave socially by observing and copying behaviour witnessed in others. These girls may also practise these behaviours further through play with dolls and toys. When taking the role of a socially skilled girl, they may re-enact scenarios and conversations they have had or overheard. This role-play helps them to analyse and rehearse situations (Attwood *et al.* 2006). The common interest of reading fiction seen in girls with autism is also a valuable tool in learning about communication and relationships. Later on in life, they may turn to psychology or self-help books for this data, but for now, Enid Blyton may well be the source of their social research. Chapter 5 on adolescence includes more about how girls with autism try to fit in by copying their peers.

> She tried to make friends by watching and copying behaviour, but it never worked particularly successfully. (Parent of girl with autism)

Mimicry is the word, although this was by no means a conscious effort. I even copy people's accents without myself knowing until the afterthought dawns on me in retrospect [...] I know I definitely was flagged a weirdo to the general populace. I guess I just didn't know. I can remember just sitting by a clique, which hopefully would not take offence to my mere presence, to pass by the more social times. (Woman with autism)

Sharing

I just did my own thing and if someone initiated conversation or wanted to play, I'd say something like, 'Sure, I'm playing with this toy, so you can play with that one'. (Woman with autism)

The notion of sharing is not always one that young children understand: 'Why would I want to give you something that leaves me with less?' The development of theory of mind at around four to six years of age usually changes this perspective and leads the child to understand that if I give you something of mine, there may be a deal here in which I can get something better in return. It is thought that children with autism develop this skill later and sometimes not to the same degree. Needing the world to be 'on their terms' is a common comment made by those living with and supporting individuals with autism. It can appear that the child is extremely self-focused, when it may be that the concept of the needs of others is simply not developed yet. This is a trait less easily tolerated in girls, who are expected to be more intuitive to the needs of others.

Sharing involves:

- Change of plan/status quo: I was doing this, now I have to adapt.

- Other people: I have no idea what they might want. It's easier to be on my own.

- Non-verbal communication: Does this person have a hidden agenda?

- Unpredictability: When will I get it back? When will it be my turn?

- Verbal negotiation: On-the-spot, socially acceptable response required.

- Anticipating the behaviour of another person.

- Sharing possessions and space: risky, loss of control and safety.

- Having to do something that you may not want to do.

It is not difficult to see why this doesn't seem like a worthwhile deal at a young age and why solo play is a more logical and low stress choice for many children with ASD. Issues with the concept of sharing were mentioned by a significant number of participants. Some did not necessarily object to it when the consequences and benefits were explained; they simply had not been aware that there was an expectation from others that it should be done.

> She finds sharing very difficult and wants everything to be done on her terms [...] 'Precious' toys have to be hidden away before other children come to play. She would never think to offer sweets to others and refuses to do so when prompted. (Woman with autism)

> I was capable of sharing, and did do it; I just didn't especially want to and didn't understand why the school didn't make adequate provision to ensure that we didn't have to share. It seemed illogical. (Woman with autism)

The differences in intuitively reading, interpreting and understanding other people that come as a core part of the autism profile mean that all people relationships are potentially fraught with stresses and misunderstandings.

Chapter 5

Adolescence

The teenage years were the worst years of my life. I was clueless to the world and felt like a fish out of water. Puberty and body changes were embarrassing and 'yuk' too.

WOMAN WITH AUTISM

Where do I begin?!

Take a socially awkward, quiet tomboy who doesn't relate to her female peers and throw a load of hormones at her. That's not going to go down well!

Puberty and adolescence are frequently a difficult time for all young women, but the combination of adolescence and autism brings it own set of challenges. Families talk about not knowing from one day to the next whether the young person's behaviour can be best explained by autism or their age (Nichols *et al.* 2009).

Friendships change, expectations change, bodies change and feelings change. It's a lot to handle for someone who takes a while to get used to change, especially when she may not be ready for these changes and just wants to carry on building Lego® and pretending to be a pony (meanwhile her classmates are swooning over some pop star and obsessing over what to wear).

> At some point in sixth grade (when I was about 11), many of the girls in my class became huggers. They hugged when they met each other and when they said goodbye. They hugged when they passed in the hallway. They hugged when they were happy or sad. They hugged and cried and squealed with excitement and I watched from

a distance, perplexed. What did all this hugging mean? And more importantly, why wasn't I suddenly feeling the need to hug someone every 30 seconds? (Kim in Hurley 2014, p.24)

On the whole, women in my survey who had been through adolescence, often without a diagnosis of autism, did not have a good word to say about this time in their lives. A few reported positively but they were often those who had successfully located a like-minded oddball or a kind neurotypical pal who gave them the acceptance that they were desperate to find; alternatively, they were the type of girl who was able to live quite happily without that acceptance.

Women were asked to describe their teenage years, and the following examples are typical of the emotions remembered:

Locked in. Caged and ultimately restricted. It's a period of my life that is a relative blur since it was so uneventful, when for most people it's a monumental time of self-discovery, exploration of the world at large and forging new directives in the way of career and life perspective etc. (Woman with autism)

I often felt as if I was peering in – looking at what others were doing, constantly observing actions and reactions. And so I learned to 'act normal'; and judging by people's reactions when I say I'm an Aspie, I'm a very good actress. (Woman with autism)

Social relationships

In the earlier years, I think I was too oblivious to social norms to notice how different I was or that I wasn't 'doing it right'. But the older I got, the more I started to feel different and anxious to be liked. (Woman with autism)

Girls with Autism Spectrum Disorder (ASD) have less severe social and communicative behaviours than boys with ASD at a young age. However, as adolescents and adults, girls have more social difficulties, particularly with peer relationships (McLennan *et al.* 1993). The prevailing view is that the peer activities commonly engaged in by girls and women are more socially and communication dependent, compared with boys, whose relationships remain largely topic- or activity-based (sport, special interests) and who, as a result, often have fewer verbal and non-verbal interpretation requirements. Rudy Simone describes this change in her own comparative social skills:

> I had many friends [...] until adolescence. All at once, my idiosyncrasies became very uncool, almost overnight. My social *deficits* [Rudy's italics], which prior to that point had just been *differences*, became glaring holes in my persona. (Simone 2010, p.28)

Stories of trying hard to fit in – and failing – were frequent in the responses. There was study, mimicry and effort involved to solve the social puzzle and gain entry into the arena of inclusion and acceptance. Liane Holliday Willey describes her own 'assimilating behaviours':

> I was uncanny in my ability to copy accents, vocal inflections, facial expressions, hand movements, gaits and tiny gestures. It was as if I became the person I was emulating. (Holliday Willey 2014, p.29)

Other difficulties arose from not only failing to understand the signals and rules governing teenage friendships, but also from the impact of making another person the object of a special interest and becoming unusually fascinated by and focused on them. The young woman with autism may seek exclusivity with the 'friend' and be confused as to why he/she would want to spend time with anyone else.

> I thought that Connie was beautiful and so clever to be able to play the piano. I followed her everywhere, and it was difficult to understand why she wanted me to go away at times, or why she wanted to be with other children and not me. (Lawson 1998, p.58)

As they get older, most girls with ASD perceive themselves as 'different' (Holliday Willey 2001; Stewart 2012), perhaps when comparing themselves directly with the social profiles of their same-gender peers. Many of the women in my sample did not receive a diagnosis until many years later, yet still recall this awareness.

I feel like I have a different operating system [with] a very good emulator running on top of it. The few people I tell are shocked to find I'm autistic. I can fit in, I can behave like others up to a point, but it isn't me and doesn't fulfil anything within me. It's empty and meaningless. (Woman with autism)

I was very aware that I was 'different' and didn't fit in and I had no wish to fit in as I couldn't see what was so great about being NT [neurotypical]. I felt rejected as my attempts to bond with peers frequently failed and I felt like my parents were ashamed of me as they thought I was weird and an embarrassment. (Woman with autism)

What also comes across from some of these women is a paradox that many people with ASD seem to struggle with: a contempt for the superficial content of the relationships of their peers, coupled with a desire to be accepted by those same peers. In the responses, there is also the relief that has come later in their adult years that they no longer have to be part of this teenage world that seemed so alien. It seems that the teenage years bring all the stress and confusion of mature social relationships but none of the adult choices of being able to opt out (due to having to endure school).

On being told by her father to 'make friends' with a girl he had introduced her to, W. Lawson describes her strategy:

She asked me lots of questions and to most of them I replied 'yes'. It seemed the safest thing to do; in my experience, when one answered 'yes' people were happier. (Lawson 1998, p.17)

I made a lot of efforts to fit in, but they all failed and by the time I was in my late teens, I'd given up. I'd known I was different since very early childhood. To be honest, these days I care very little about fitting in. I see the NT world and culture for what it is and I have little interest in selling out to be a part of it. (Woman with autism)

I tried to wear the right clothes or be interested in things others were to fit in but I never quite pulled it off. It's a bit like trying to speak another language that I'm not fluent in – I can get by for so long but eventually I'm always found out and my ignorance is revealed. (Woman with autism)

Opinions on social relationships, particularly with other girls, are a clear indicator that these young women thought and felt differently to their peers. They had different agendas, different interests and different requirements from a friendship. Some were bullied, some were excluded and some were permitted to exist on the fringes.

Girls in real life are not something I enjoy being near, especially loud, squealy, hair-and-make-up high-schoolers. (Woman with autism)

One time, aged 13 a girl did an experiment on me by calling me a bitch. I was confused because she was one of the few who was normally nice to me, or at least not horrid, and then she said, 'You don't know how to react do you?' She'd clearly noticed that I simply did not have a response in my repertoire to such things. (Woman with autism)

Others seemed not to rankle and engender the displeasure of their female peers, either by being invisible and/or of no interest, or by being endearing and tolerated to some degree.

As a teen I was quite lucky – I was 'allowed' to hang onto the edges of two girls who had been best friends since they were young. (Woman with autism)

I was a tomboy, did not get into make-up, but wished I could be more like the other girls. I loved motorbikes, got one and learned how to take it apart and fix it. (Woman with autism)

For young women today, the Internet appears to offer a space for developing friendships based on interests and not requiring the complexities of face-to-face interaction – no-one cares if you're wearing the right clothes or not making the right facial expressions. Some younger women said that all of their interactions were Internet-based and that they had no in-person social contact at all. Video-gaming was important to several of the younger respondents, and their involvement in these communities had provided them with friends.

> I have friends on the Internet. They are a mix of male and female, and points in-between. I talk to them on a varying basis, always one-to-one. I would like more friends, but I do not wish to burden them. (Woman with autism)

The additional expectations of young women with autism in terms of social ability, self-care, education and independence may lead to more visible mental health difficulties during this time. They may develop obvious signs of anxiety, self-harm or eating disorders, which may not be linked with autism by professionals as this may not have been diagnosed yet. Some of these behaviours can be incorrectly attributed simply to puberty and treated in a way that does not address the underlying stress involved in living with autism.

> As a teenager and young adult I did what was expected of me in order to fit in. I went to night clubs, which I hated. I went to guide camp, which made me ill as I was so distressed. Even after that I went on holiday to Spain with a school friend just because it was the expected thing to do. I came home half-way though and spent about a year recovering as my mental health was affected so badly. (Woman with autism)

> It feels lonely, but at the same time, I know I should never burden people with my issues, and that I should tackle everything alone. If anything, it's the only way I can prove myself to be as good as anyone else. (Woman with autism, aged 18 years)

Characteristics

Some of the typical diagnostic characteristics of ASD can be less obvious as a girl gets older – this may particularly apply to more intellectually able and self-aware individuals who learn what is required and what is deemed unacceptable. Young women with autism, as we have heard, are often excellent social anthropologists, studying the behaviours of others in order to predict more accurately what neurotypicals will do, and also to imitate this behaviour themselves in order to receive either social approval, or at the very least, slip under the radar to some degree. They are not always entirely successful and their experiences can alert us to what we should be looking for in undiagnosed young women.

Communication and social understanding

> I was only taught how to make eye contact soon after I turned 17. Before that, because I didn't know the correct way, I would simply avoid doing it. (Woman with autism)

> Socially, I suspect I came across as cold and aloof to people, which is a shame as I'm not like that, but I don't pull the faces and do the gestures that NTs are so taken with, so I am judged negatively before people even bother to get to know me. (Woman with autism)

> My teens were full of 'what you f**king looking at?' by other girls. This was incredibly confusing and frightening to me. Obviously something in my facial expression was upsetting them, but I really don't know what. (Woman with autism)

Interests

Intense interests exist throughout the lifetime of people with ASD, but they can change and develop with age. For young women in my sample, reading still featured heavily, as it had done when they were children. Drawing, writing, sewing and collecting were all reported. The interests mentioned are solitary pursuits and no-one mentioned sharing these interests with peers (other than video-gaming, which was remote interaction rather than in the same room). People still formed a significant part of the young women's interests, either through fictional characters or obsessions or crushes on people known to them. The solitary nature of these interests could lead to the assumption of shyness, isolation, depression or social anxiety – all of which may be the case, but which, equally, may mask underlying autism.

I was into music big time. I preferred music from before my day and disliked the stuff my peers were into. During my teens I liked rock and roll music from the 50s and 60s and would play my favourite tracks over and over again; I knew all the words and all about the artists. (Woman with autism)

In my teens I was obsessed with the Royal Navy. Then I think my obsessions were mostly people – partners and the future I hoped to build with them. I also spent several years obsessed by cricket, both playing and watching. (Woman with autism)

I have spent much of my teenage and adult years reading fiction, playing computer games and watching fiction on TV. Many times I've felt closer to fictional characters than real-life people. (Woman with autism)

Coping with change

I came home to find we had a new sofa and the old one was outside in the yard. Again I went mad and went and sat on the old one in the yard, claiming I was going to live outside. Again I didn't understand my reaction, but it was very strong and I was horrible to my mum about it. (Woman with autism)

Despite being often outwardly capable, most of the women I asked reported life-long issues with changes to plans and routines. As teenagers, these could result in outbursts and an anxious need for reassurance or detail, which may be attributed to typical teenage behaviour, but with hindsight, may be explicable through the lens of autism. Even small changes to environments or plans could cause enormous stress that the young woman with autism would not be able to articulate or put into perspective at this time in her life. Anecdotally, it is often reported that women with autism are more likely to internalise the anxiety and stress they feel around change, not wanting to draw attention to their inability to cope with the situation. This leads other people to believe that they are coping, when in fact they are not. Repression of emotions and the effort involved in hiding them from others can cause long-term mental health problems, and eventually the facade crashes as the curtailed stress has to come out.

Independent skills

Many of these young women were extremely capable and independent, further masking their potential difficulties. They usually behaved well and did what was asked of them to the letter, being seen as very mature and sensible. Adults tend to like children who behave like little adults, perhaps not appreciating that a child behaving in this way is not always a good thing!

> I was conscientious and responsible. (Woman with autism)

> I see the world as a puzzle to be solved, and meticulous planning means I function well, though with more stress. (Woman with autism)

> I manage by means of a complex schedule and a series of lists. My short-term memory is terrible and without this, I would not be able to function. (Woman with autism)

Others found expectations of their abilities impossible to meet, sometimes hiding these difficulties and finding their own ways to cope.

> I struggled to cope with public transport and used to walk the two miles each way to school rather than get the bus. I don't know why I found it difficult – probably just the compulsory interaction with the bus driver and my peers on the bus. I just couldn't cope with it. I was allowed so little time alone that the 40-minute walk to school and back, alone, was a relief. (Woman with autism)

Periods and puberty

Understanding and knowledge about matters involving physical and hormonal changes during puberty may be more limited in this group of girls due to their potentially limited peer group, which is typically the main source of this information for most young people. Support to ensure that young women with autism receive this information and have the opportunity to ask questions is essential. Shana Nichols *et al.* (2009) have written *Girls Growing Up on the Autism Spectrum*, a comprehensive guide to supporting girls in dealing with all issues relating to puberty and adolescence. Witnessing your own body changing without any understanding of what is happening can lead to anxiety and fear about something that is perfectly normal. A girl with autism may not feel able to talk to anyone about her worries as she may be afraid that there is something wrong with her.

> At about the age of 11, I found a magazine in the newsagents called the *Mizz Book of Love*. This magazine was a treasure trove of factual info about puberty, sex, STI [sexually transmitted infection], pregnancy etc. Thank God I found this magazine. I was not shocked at puberty because I knew what to expect; in fact, I was excited and happy to change into a woman. I am certain that educating young girls on the spectrum in depth is essential. I already discuss the facts of life, including sex abuse, with my six-year-old daughter – she can ask me anything and I will tell her. I feel very strongly about this. She needs to know. (Woman with autism)

> I was 12 when my periods started and I hated it with a passion. Mum hadn't told me anything about them and I didn't have other girls to tell me, although the school did a talk about it. During the talk I was pretty horrified at what I was hearing and I think I prevented myself from taking it in. I remember they passed round a sanitary towel and I refused to touch it. I think I concluded that 'No thank you, this stuff wasn't going to happen to me!' (Woman with autism)

Keeping clean, changing sanitary protection and avoid embarrassing mishaps are skills that may need to be taught to young women reaching puberty. Liane Holliday Willey (2012) describes her frequent 'accidents' with forgetting to change tampons, resulting in blood stains on furniture. Some young women don't know when they should start to wear a bra or how to have that conversation with their parents or carers. Wearing a bra takes some getting used to, particularly if you have sensory sensitivity to touch. It can be unbearably uncomfortable. Nichols *et al.* (2009) discuss the issue of bras and how to address the concept. Some women with autism continue into adulthood choosing not to wear a bra, which is a personal right, but one that comes with potential consequences. I worked with a young woman with very large breasts who did not see why she should wear a bra, but was not aware that her bosom was very obvious and that people stared at her and made negative comments. Her decision may also have had implications for her physical health as she had no support for her breasts and her back. The decision was hers to make, but she needed to have honest advice about other people's perceptions and any health implications in order to enable her to make an informed choice. This was to continue to not wear a bra as she didn't care what people thought. Some women with autism do not wish to conform to societal norms that they feel do not fit them and should be supported to do so once they know all the consequences.

Hygiene is another area that takes on greater importance from the onset of puberty, with some young women with autism not really understanding or being concerned about the health and social impacts of being dirty and smelling bad. The consequences and actual skills of self-care may need to be taught in detail. It cannot be assumed that the individual with autism knows how much shampoo to use, how to rinse it out and what the purpose of deodorant is.

> Still not great with personal hygiene, I mostly wash in order to stop getting sore or so that other people don't think I'm stinky. Being stinky doesn't really worry me. (Woman with autism)

Overall, we can conclude that the teenage years are a time of enormous change, development and learning for young women with autism. All young people find these years difficult at times but the social exclusion and changing nature of friendships, along with increased expectations from families and teachers, mean that young women with autism are faced with additional challenges.

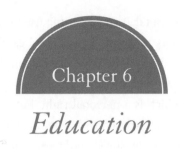

Chapter 6

Education

Despite a love of learning and an appetite for information, Aspergirls do not all enjoy school the way others might think that they would.

SIMONE (2010, P.27)

At the risk of stating the obvious, a child spends a large proportion of their waking hours at school. School is not home. School does not have Mum/Dad/carer/family in it. Nor does it have a perfectly colour-co-ordinated, unplayed-with collection of My Little Ponies, or X-Men, for that matter. School has people in it: lots of them. As Rudy Simone puts it, 'Most of the Aspergirls said the same thing […] school was boring and they were bullied' (2010, p.27).

For the child with Autism Spectrum Disorder (ASD) school constitutes a lack of control in all aspects of their world and hence can be a place of great trauma and anxiety. It is a constantly social environment. It can also be a place of knowledge, usefulness and structure. The extent to which the experience is positive or negative for the child is often a result of the understanding of her ASD by those in authority and their willingness to help her out. For girls, the aforementioned late, or non-existent, diagnosis and limited understanding of the female presentation ('She's quiet: she's fine') can mean that the school experience is often far from positive, as we shall hear. Eileen Riley-Hall, in her book *Parenting Girls on the Autism Spectrum* (2012), presents a whole chapter outlining education options and processes in both the US and the UK, which covers the practicalities and considerations with far more skill than I can here.

As we progress through this book and look at adult outcomes for women with ASD, we will see that intelligence does not necessarily lead to a conventionally successful outcome. Many women with ASD have to find their own rocky path to their own version of success, which may come later and in a different form to anything anyone could have predicted from that bright, quiet, bookworm of a girl.

On the whole, the girls and women with ASD who participated in the research for this book – particularly those diagnosed in adulthood – had a rotten time in their school years due to a lack of early diagnosis, support and any understanding of their perception of the school experience. This knowledge is useful in enabling us to identify how they felt and what went wrong for them and to put measures in place to prevent other girls with ASD from having the same experiences. This is a hope shared by one mother for her daughter:

> It was a long road to get A recognised as being on the spectrum. Once support is in place, the difference is remarkable; I am almost envious and wish that I had had this understanding. It is my mission that she will not end up like me. Her home will be her haven, she will find love, understanding and support from her parents and I will insist that her school does the same. All of her desires and interests are supported; I cannot bear the thought of her feeling frustrated like I did. I look back and wonder what I could have been had my interests been indulged. (Mother with autism, who has a daughter with autism)

It is sometimes not until a child begins some form of formal education that their ASD starts to become apparent. All children have their own quirks and preferences, which are met and managed within the home and the family, and it may not be until the child is required to tolerate a large number of other children plus a few strangers for several hours a day that problems arise. She may have been an active helper to her mother at home, polite and talkative to visitors, relaxed and outgoing with her family and happy organising her toys and collections; a child who shows no signs of visible stress, because there probably wasn't any. When asked about their experiences of their children starting pre-school, parents report:

> Starting school was awful. Up until this time she was a happy, lovely little girl. The anxiety she feels is very upsetting. To be honest, I think she has resigned herself to school. I will consider home school when she is older if she finds it too difficult; the damage it could cause her is something I know only too well. (Parent of girl with autism)

> Dreadful. It was then that we started to really see the differences. (Parent of girl with autism)

Some children have no concept of why they are going to this new place. It may seem obvious to us that this is simply 'the way things are' after a certain age, but this assumption cannot be made for a child with ASD. We may assume that the socialising aspect of play settings is beneficial to the child. This is an almost universally held belief, particularly in the case of girls. The child with ASD may disagree. It may be that for some children with ASD there really is no point or functional benefit in them attending a group play setting and that the distress caused outweighs any possible benefit gained. This notion is difficult for many parents to acknowledge as they believe that being alone cannot be good for the child; but for many children and adults with ASD, being alone is the best thing of all.

> I was distraught and in tears and didn't want to go. I didn't see the point. I would regularly vomit in the car on the way to pre-school. (Woman with autism)

Capacity can become stretched for the first time in the child's life and very different behaviours may be observed. For the child herself, the world has suddenly changed beyond all recognition and has potentially become very frightening; she has had to leave her home (her sanctuary) and in its place there is this cacophonous, labyrinthine, stranger-filled abyss. In the responses to my questions, there was a marked difference between those who were diagnosed in adulthood, who had to navigate school without a label or any adjustments, and those who are still children with a diagnosis and receiving support (although this may have been hard fought for by their parents and initially traumatic for the child).

> The transition to pre-school was very difficult. She became upset and didn't want to go in [...] The manager asked me to stay every day for three weeks and then I gradually stayed for less and less time. [The manager] said that she had never had a child who reacted like this for such a long time. The transition to primary school was much better. We knew that she probably had autism at this stage, and a comprehensive transition plan was put into place. She settled in quickly and enjoyed it. (Parent of girl with autism)

Eileen Riley-Hall (2012) advises parents to take a photograph of their daughter to any meeting to discuss her education in order to remind everyone present that she 'is a person, not just a program to be created in a cost-effective manner' (p.49).

The adult-diagnosed women's recollections are, in the vast majority of cases, negative and painful to read: 'dreadful', 'awful', 'horrific', 'distraught' are the words they use. For parents of children who have managed to get support in place, the story is remarkably different and positive. Comparing these experiences lends huge hope and support to the idea that knowledge and a change in attitude can make a real difference for the daily experience of the child with autism. The tales of late-diagnosed women give insight into a world that we should not be subjecting a child with ASD to in the present day.

> I remember early on [...] crying and hiding behind a door when we walked from one classroom to a new classroom and I was unaware of what was going to happen. (Woman with autism)

> My mum says I hated nursery. She never managed to leave me there for a full day as the teachers often had to call her because I was crying so much. (Woman with autism)

Horrific, traumatic experience, which sadly never improved. (Woman with autism)

The school environment was stressful and hectic and full of people who seemed to hate me for no reason. (Woman with autism)

Many of the comments and experiences here could apply to both boys and girls, but some are more indicative of the female profile and of others' expectations of girls' behaviour and social abilities, which these girls may not be able (or aspire) to match up to. It is difficult to convey just how deep-seated and a core part of society these gender expectations are, and how hard it is to consciously recognise these girls and be willing to view them as different but equally acceptable just as they are.

There are many books on educating children on the autism spectrum, with tips, tools and techniques that go into great depth. I will touch on a few here, but my main purpose is to illustrate the female experience in a school setting. The intention is not to frighten professionals or parents of young girls with ASD into seeing the horrors that lie ahead; rather, it is to prevent these experiences happening to future generations of girls. The headings below are not consistent across each educational setting as different aspects cause different levels of difficulty at different stages. I would advise that reading through all settings might be worthwhile to get a picture of potential issues in education as a whole rather than just isolating one age group. Any child or adult with whom you are working will either have already experienced much of what is discussed through these sections, or has yet to do so as they move forward through the education system. Either way, a holistic consideration of the impact of their past and potential future should enable any professional to better consider appropriate educational measures to be put in place.

Early Years – pre-school, nursery and playgroup

Physical environment

This is a young girl's first experience of spending significant time with people other than her family and in an unfamiliar environment. In the UK, these Early Years experiences may sometimes take place in a building that is not built as a place of learning and that is used for many functions throughout the day – a church hall, Scout hut or leisure centre, for example. The rooms are often large, old and have strange acoustics. Furniture and equipment have to be set out and packed away at the start and end of each session and that can mean that materials and space may be limited and not very adaptable. The impact of these factors on a child with autism may be that they experience stress around the sensory environment in terms of noise and acoustics, but also in terms of a lack of consistency about the layout of the space. I have worked with children (and adults) who cannot tolerate furniture being moved in a classroom without their presence; for them it is like entering an entirely different place and requires them to entirely reconfigure their understanding of where they are every time they enter the room. Something as simple as this could result in anxiety and so-called 'challenging behaviour'.

Teaching and support staff

Early Years settings are often partly staffed by volunteers, who may have limited or no knowledge or experience of ASD – particularly as it is often not diagnosed in this age group unless there are significant verbal or global developmental indicators. In contrast, they may have plenty of knowledge about how they expect a neurotypical child of this age to behave. These general expectations of what is typical can put pressure on the child to conform in ways that are unmanageably difficult for them, but nobody knows why they become so distressed. A requirement to sit on an itchy carpet, touch wet sand or hold hands with another child may make the setting unbearable for a child with ASD.

> They insisted on tying my hair up and I found this very painful. Until recently when I read about autistic people having scalp sensitivity,

I blamed them for being horrid and pulling my hair so painfully. (Woman with autism)

Training and awareness for staff working in these settings is crucial in ensuring early positive experiences for young girls with ASD, even if the ASD is only suspected by the parent at this stage. Diagnosis is unlikely to have taken place for many of these girls at this age, but early signs of difference should be accommodated, regardless of official recognition. It may only be possible to make limited adjustments to the environment due to factors outside the Early Years organiser's control, but small measures can make a huge difference; a quiet space being made available with headphones, being permitted to hold a teacher's belt rather than her hand, wearing rubber gloves while playing in the sand pit, a beanbag and a favourite toy are strategies that might provide a small respite and reduce anxiety for a child who is feeling overwhelmed or overloaded.

Communication and structure

Early Years settings can be quite fluid and flexible in their schedules, which may cause additional difficulties for the child with ASD who does not know what is going to happen unless explicitly told. Some children become distressed at their parent leaving them at playgroup or school because no-one informed them that the parent would return. Without the benefit of imagination, the child may assume that she will never see her parent again, which makes the level of distress understandable in that context.

Some level of predictability and timetabling might help a child with autism to cope with knowing what to expect each day and how and when it will start and end. Explicit and visual reassurance can support the child in managing her own anxious feelings.

At playgroup, she seemed to find unstructured play unsettling. Was often telling the adults that they were wrong, e.g., spelling or simple facts (usually correctly!). Was seen as aloof and a bit posh! (Parent of girl with autism)

A pictorial schedule of the day pinned to the wall might provide evidence of certainty and the child can be encouraged to learn where to find the information she needs on it. This may also give the child the chance to look forward to certain activities and encourage her to attend – particularly if these can be tailored to meet the child's interests. Being told that tomorrow she will be able to look at pictures of cats and draw cats – if cats are her 'thing' – may help a reluctant child to feel motivated to attend. In terms of other motivators, it may be that social ones don't work. As we shall see below, other children were often the cause of difficulty and apprehension about attending school or nursery. Attempting to persuade a girl with ASD to go to playgroup in order to 'play with her friends' might remind her of the horror of sharing toys and reduce her to tears and panic. For many children with ASD, free playtime is the hardest time of all to manage. Identifying the motivators that are meaningful to her – interests, favourite carer, specific toys, biscuits at breaktime and chocolate on the journey home if she makes it through the day – is most likely to achieve success.

School

The transition from an Early Years setting into school can be quite a shock for a child with ASD. A uniform with all of its required sensory tolerance may be insisted upon; the length of the school day may increase two-fold and the afternoon nap is a thing of the past. Although some children with ASD embrace the clear rules, structure and boundaries that school imposes, since these things provide routine and hence a sense of safety and relief, others find the number of people and the length of the school day extremely difficult to manage. Good preparation for this, prior to the child starting school, is essential to ensure that the child understands what school involves and has some idea of the environment that she will be spending her days in.

> She finds school emotionally draining [...] she would often 'explode' the minute she left the school gate and I learned that it was best not to

speak to her at all while we walked home because any conversation would lead to meltdown. (Parent of girl with autism)

It is necessary to remember that the girl with ASD may not appear to have any difficulties; she may be the ideal child, helpful and polite. This may be the case at first, but as she gets older and additional demands are made of her, both socially and educationally, the mask may start to slip. (It has been shown that increased demands in both of these areas contribute to increased anxiety in girls with ASD (Stewart 2012)). And, as we have seen, when the mask slips, something that looks like mental health issues can be revealed; however, careful observation may lead to the conclusion that changes in a girl's behaviour are simply the result of an inability to maintain the neurotypical persona that she has learned to create.

An important thing to note, and that has been seen in this research and elsewhere (e.g., Stewart 2012), is that girls with ASD want to do well, comply and not get into trouble. As professionals, if we always keep in mind that when a girl is doing something that on the face of it appears rude, diffident or downright obstructive, she is, in fact, trying her hardest to do the right thing, regardless of how it might appear, we can support her by understanding what she is trying to say or do and teach her a new way of doing it in the future.

Breaktimes and social interaction

For many children with ASD, breaktime is the most difficult part of the school day. The structure of the lessons is gone and the entire population of the school is released into the playground, our girl included. Suddenly, social abilities reign supreme and an understanding of the complexities of relationships, negotiation and rules of play is required. It would be fair to say that our girl with ASD may well return to the classroom after a 'break' more exhausted than she was when she left it. This is an extremely important point and one that must be considered in reflecting on behaviour, performance and general well-being at school.

[The playground] was noisy, unorganised chaos. I went home for lunches and avoided busy [areas] at playtime. (Woman with autism)

I wanted to stay in and read a book, but was not allowed. I spent most playtimes alone. (Woman with autism)

I would stand by the punishment wall (a place where kids were sent to stand if they had done bad things) every playtime of every day, and do nothing but stand there during that time. (Woman with autism)

Playtime remains difficult for A. We asked the school to give her more supervision, access to a quiet area indoors, a place for her to eat her lunch outside the dining hall at times of high anxiety as these things are very hard for her. (Parent of girl with autism)

As girls get older, their friendships change, and they move away from toy-based, pretence games to more sophisticated people and personality-based relationships. Girls talk about other girls (and boys); their relationships are subtle and nuanced, and allegiances are forever changing. Girls with ASD struggle increasingly with age to, first understand why this change has occurred – they were quite happy as things were – and, second to be able to continue to hold their own in this new social arena (Riley-Hall 2012). School breaktime is the primary location for this new terror – and it happens three times a day. This is supposed to be the part of the day that is 'fun'! For parents, the expectation may be that seeing friends after school is a natural thing for their child to want to do. The parent of one girl explains beautifully the perspective of her daughter with regard to socialising after school:

We rarely had playdates in the first couple of years because she said, 'I've been at school with people all day – why would I want to see them again now?' (Parent of girl with autism)

Learning and teaching style

Many of the women and girls who participated in this book were precocious early talkers, often with extensive vocabularies. This does not mean that learning came/comes easily to them, on account of the neurotypical system they were/are expected to adhere to. We must not forget that, even in a learning environment, social requirements are always present, which means that our girl with ASD has to work doubly hard to make sense of both the social and the academic elements.

> I had little interest in other children and would much rather have been left alone with books to study by myself or just have one-to-one lessons. Being around the other children was a huge impediment to my learning, well-being and mental health. (Woman with autism)

> Due to my constant daydreaming and struggles following spoken instructions, I had a lot of trouble with learning. (Woman with autism)

> I was pretty good academically; my biggest difficulty was probably with my own arrogance and I felt I was superior to not only the other kids but to the teacher. (Woman with autism)

We know that individuals with ASD find life easier if there is some structure and predictability about what's coming next. It means that anxiety is reduced and therefore the capacity and ability for learning are increased. School is often full of rituals, routines and structures. Unfortunately, many of these make little sense as they may have a social or compliance basis rather than a logical one. They may also be imposed without any contextual explanation to enable the child to learn why these social behaviours are beneficial and/or necessary. Being reprimanded for doing something that you didn't know you had to do and why you had to do it – and hence are unlikely to understand the context of when to do it next time – causes anxiety. Knowing that you will undoubtedly get something 'wrong', but are not sure what or when, is perhaps why children with ASD can develop school phobia.

It is thought that girls with ASD are more likely to suffer in silence (Wagner 2006) and that their 'shy' profile means their learning difficulties go unnoticed. These girls may just be seen as poorly performing students. The desire to fit in and not be seen as stupid by their peers may explain a reluctance to raise their hands to answer a question or to stand out in any way.

> She is a perfectionist [...] she would not put up her hand or answer a question for many years in case she was wrong [...] She generally sits at the back saying very little but still manages to produce excellent work. (Parent of girl with autism)

> She won't speak to a teacher because she 'doesn't want to bother them' and 'might get shouted at'. This is a problem because she will never ask if she doesn't understand. (Parent of girl with autism)

Subjects

Among those women questioned, art and English topped the list of favourite subjects at school. These are not the typically expected 'male' ASD topics (usually involving maths and IT), which may add to the difficulty in considering an ASD diagnosis for a literary and creative girl. Many were voracious readers and most happy when engrossed in a book during the school day. They also enjoyed drawing and colouring – perceived as typical female pursuits. Gathering factual (or fictional) information in a solo world appears to be more enjoyable than gathering social information in the real world for these girls, and their knowledge of chosen subjects can be extensive. My personal experience was of being constantly described as 'lazy' by teachers for never achieving an 'A' grade despite being a gifted-level student with precocious early speech. I have always said that I knew the answer, but I didn't know the question. It was other people's language I had trouble with, not my own. Language processing (verbal and written) made much of learning inaccessible, but I was fortunate to be able to scrape through using intellect and logic, which has its limitations. This remains the same in my adult life.

Girls with ASD, like their male peers, can show unusual, uneven learning profiles, where instead of having a fairly consistent profile of ability, they exhibit extreme subject area peaks and troughs. The causes of this can be a combination of:

- the cognitive profile of autism itself

- the nature of the subject being taught

- the individual's natural processing style and ability

- the teaching style

- the level of interest and motivation that the student has in the topic.

All or some of these elements can combine to create a greater or lesser ability in certain subjects. If the subject content is inaccessible, due to either its nature or the way in which it is taught, a student with ASD is more likely to switch off and feel incapable of engaging. The logical nature of those with ASD leads some to conclude that if they know they are going to fail at something, why bother to even try?

> I saw little point in doing any subject I wasn't good at as it seemed a waste of time and just an exercise in futility and self-humiliation. (Woman with autism)

Something as simple as considering a different teaching approach or explaining a broader contextual reason for the purpose of the topic can bring about a change in attitude and performance in certain subjects.

Teaching staff

Research has shown that teachers are less likely to notice and/or report difficulties with adapting in girls with autism than boys (Mandy *et al.* 2012), perhaps due to the invisible presentation in girls and the perception of ASD as a male condition. Girls with ASD have been found to exhibit less restricted, stereotyped behaviours, which are a known visible sign of potential ASD. It may well be that if a teacher does not notice any such behaviour, they may not be open to the possibility of ASD. Teachers rarely have sufficient knowledge of autism, even less so its presentation in girls (Wagner 2006). Constant misunderstandings from teachers were a common theme in the responses of my participants and have also been identified as a concern elsewhere. Catriona Stewart states that:

As they worked to establish a system of rules that allowed them to function (i.e. systems of behaviour relating to logic, sustainability, cause and effect, predictable outcomes, fairness), the girls were expected to function in a world of people whose behaviour did not adhere to them. (Stewart 2012, p.42)

I did well in school but did not speak a lot and ended up in detention for really [trival] things like not talking. (Woman with autism)

She tells me how she was sent to the Principal's office because she had kicked someone under the table. She says she didn't know why she was there or what she had done – she was just swinging her legs. (Parent of girl with autism)

We were playing a game where everyone stands in a line with their feet apart, and the person at the front rolls a ball through everyone's legs to be caught by the last person in the line, who runs to the front [...] The teacher pulled me out of the line and shook me in front of everyone, and I never did understand what for. (Woman with autism)

Teachers are predominantly female and perhaps, given their people-focused, flexible, communication-based career choice, may be quite different in personality from their young, female charges with ASD. When one considers the difficulties that these girls can have with their female peers, it shouldn't surprise us that they have similar problems with the grown-up versions of those peers, who may become teachers! It is also important to remember that relationships are reciprocal, so it is not simply the case that the girl with ASD doesn't understand and relate well to her more intuitively communicative teacher; it is equally the case that the teacher may not feel that she has 'connected' with this unusual (especially so for a 'girl') child. The standard reciprocal 'positive strokes' may not be there and the teacher may be confused by their feelings about this girl. Children with ASD may also be highly knowledgeable in certain subjects and, not perceiving the invisible social rules of hierarchy, may quite confidently correct or interject when a teacher is speaking. This can be perceived as a deliberate attempt at insult by a teacher, whereas the girl is simply presenting empirical facts and has no agenda to cause emotional harm or any understanding that she may be doing so.

As professionals, it is essential that people self-reflect and separate their – often strong – personal feelings towards a person from their professional duty to do the right thing for that individual. I am not aware that teacher training programmes include this type of practice, but it is my belief that they should. It may be that the teacher is not even aware of why this child upsets them so much as it can occur on an subconscious level. People who are very emotionally intuitive can sometimes take the behaviour of this type of girl personally and assume that she is deliberately trying to make life difficult. The insights from girls and women with ASD reveal that this is seldom, if ever, the case. Mostly, they are desperate to get it right and gain approval and acceptance, but despite their best efforts, they often appear to do the one thing that causes a teacher to react very badly to them at times.

> They [teachers] didn't like me, thought I was lazy, and often accused me [of] being an attention-seeker, when all I really did was actually avoid everyone. (Woman with autism)

> Some [teachers] felt her rude/insolent when she showed high levels of knowledge and intelligence. (Parent of girl with autism)

> They [teachers] seemed to think I was choosing to be different and to have social difficulties [...] One teacher bullied me terribly and used to reprimand me for not giving him eye contact. (Woman with autism)

It is worth noting that there is often an expectation that girls will be better than boys at social niceties and so may be judged differently – and sometimes more harshly – when they fail to behave in a 'nice' way on occasions where their intentions may have been misinterpreted. The following is a good example of this:

> I wanted to surprise my friend by taking her outside and getting her to feel the rain in her face. She was still in the classroom so I covered her eyes and took her out of the class, walking blindly while

telling her it was a surprise. As we walked down onto the patio she tripped, fell on a muddy patch, and her uniform got dirty. A teacher noticed and came over. She called me a 'nasty, ugly girl'. I was not given the chance to explain, nor had I the verbal skills to interrupt and explain what I had intended to do. I had had no malicious intent whatsoever. (Woman with autism)

Physical environment

For a lot of school, we sat alone at desks, not in groups. This was perfect for me. (Woman with autism)

For many young women with ASD, the physical environment of mainstream school is extremely stressful (Stewart 2012) and this gets worse as they grow older. School dining halls are notoriously overwhelming for children with ASD, mainly because of the noise (cutlery, scraping chairs, banging plates, incessant chatter) but also because of the smell, visual overload and social elements (where shall I sit?). This stress can be exacerbated when there is the requirement to navigate the complex female social world of working out allegiances and non-verbal signals. One girl did not eat at lunchtime because the dining area was intolerable for her (Stewart 2012), leading to potential health issues.

Education in adolescence and beyond

The main problem for young women with autism at school during the teenage years is their social relationships and ability to be around other people for extended periods of time. The challenges of earlier childhood school remain but are exacerbated by an increased awareness of the difference between them and their peers. Spending time surrounded by teenagers at school is a constant reminder of these feelings of difference, and it is unavoidable.

I was totally lost as a teen at school, I had no idea how to pull off fitting in and didn't want to be like the others. I wanted school to be about learning exciting, interesting stuff and then the subject matter being what everyone talked about, but alas that wasn't the case. School seemed to be one big social experience and the learning and subject matter were irrelevant to most people. (Woman with autism)

When things were fine the autism helped my education – memory, numerical skill etc. But when things went wrong people were quick to judge things as 'hormonal/emotional problems' or 'attention seeking' rather than listen to me try to explain the actual issues. (Woman with autism)

Sharing space was a problem. I didn't care to be around others much and during the teenage years – at school, home and work – I was trapped with people, which was horrendous for me. I used to spend ages in the bathroom with the door locked as it was the only place I could be alone with my thoughts. (Woman with autism)

College

I had convinced myself that my high IQ and high academic achievement record meant I was strong enough to handle whatever came my way [...] I was hit hard when I had to realise smarts were not enough to make it in this world. I was turned upside down when I had to admit I could not find anyone who saw things like I did. (Liane Holliday Willey 2014, p.63)

Liane writes of how she had an accepting group of friends at school and how she expected to find the same at college, but instead found herself floundering in a bigger, unknown environment. While being bullied often decreases as people get older, it can be replaced with invisibility, which feels like rejection, regardless of intent. College means starting over again, with the need to initiate new relationships, but these are more adult, and more socially nuanced than the last time that this had to be done at the start of school.

Some women in my survey found that college was easier than school as there is more freedom of movement, there are fewer classes per day and you are able to choose to study subjects that you excel at and enjoy. The more mature treatment of students at college suits some individuals with autism – those who like control and autonomy, and simply to be left alone. A few found kindred spirits in their tutors, who offered knowledge and an escape.

> I found it much easier to deal with college. When you are at school you cannot be alone at lunch/breaktimes, but at college it's seen as quite acceptable to go to the library, or study or sit quietly and read a book. (Woman with autism)

> I spent a considerable amount of time chatting to one of my lecturers, who was, on reflection, obviously on the [autism] spectrum [...] If it wasn't for him, I don't think I would have achieved my A-levels. His office was like a sanctuary for me. (Woman with autism)

University

The challenges of university for women with autism are largely similar to those of men with autism, and other writing focuses on these aspects in greater detail. For women, the specific difficulties remain the same as for other areas of life: social interaction with female peers, mental health problems as a result of difficulties coping with what is required of them and lack of diagnosis, and, therefore, lack of understanding or support of any kind. The key to a successful experience of university appears for many young women to be linked to social integration and acceptance. They may have the academic abilities to undertake the work, but the isolation and implicit rejection can make the difference between successful completion and dropping out. Personal relationship issues are discussed elsewhere, but might also be a contributory factor during this time.

> When I went to university, I failed my first year. The other students were girly girls; I just did not fit in. I felt very lonely and missed tons of lectures and deadlines. They failed me but allowed me to re-sit the year [...] Thankfully, I got together with a group of students.

We were a bunch of misfits [...] We had a great time – those three years were brilliant. I felt completely accepted in my circle of friends and successfully completed my degree, with a few deadline extensions! (Woman with autism)

I'm doing a distance learning course, so I don't really have to interact much with people. The occasional presentation or Skype discussion I can cope with, although I'm very self-conscious about these and find them stressful. (Woman with autism)

My autism wasn't diagnosed until after university. I feel that had I been a male child, it would have been picked up sooner [...] At university, I was mentally ill and I struggled to cope socially too as I don't drink and I don't go to clubs or pubs. I didn't speak to anyone other than my tutors for the first year and nearly left on several occasions. When I tried to interact with people or be open about my difficulties and distress, people just became exasperated and bored with me, like I was a nuisance rather than someone desperate for support. (Woman with autism)

Educational support

Although every girl and young woman with autism will need an individualised support plan to meet her needs, there are a number of general approaches teachers can adopt that will certainly aid the child's process of transition and settling into a new educational setting:

- Put the support in place before she starts at your school.

- Meet her before she starts, show her around – let her know where she will be and what's required. Find her a pal to help her find her way into the social side of things.

- Use visuals, schedules and other concrete information to help her settle in and make sense of what will happen and when.

- Girls with ASD generally want to do well, comply and stay out of trouble. If this is not happening, the chances are she has a gap in her understanding of what's required. Remember this before reacting.

- Do not take what she says or does personally. She is not meaning to annoy you. (If she is unable to predict the thoughts and feelings of others, she won't have a clue how to wind you up.)

- Consider your rules. Are you and others adhering to them? She will be – sometimes in a very literal and black-and-white way. The rules that she has been given may be all she has to navigate the world. The fact that others don't appear to have to stick to them will distress and confuse her greatly.

- Staff need training in ASD and specifically how it manifests in girls.

- Don't assume that because she's smart (or average) she will be fine. She won't. All the qualifications in the world don't mean a thing if you can't hold a conversation.

- Teach the non-academic skills – even if you have a doctorate, you still need to be able to answer a phone or make the tea. She may not be able to do either of these things.

- Consider language processing limitations – just because she is highly articulate (her words) doesn't mean that she can comprehend what you require (your words). One does not equal the other – often it is completely the opposite. She is literal and eloquent purely because it's the one and only way that she understands the concept.

- Pre-teach the content of lessons. Give her the heads-up on the topic area in advance and let her go and research it on her own. In this way, she will have had time to process the information, reducing surprises and increasing her ability to participate in the lessons. Do this with all your students.

- Ensure that she understands the requirements of assignments. Provide her with parameters and guidelines on length, content, timescale and priority so that she doesn't spend too long striving for perfection when it's not necessary.

- Keep an eye on her. She may not ask for help. Asking for help may equate to weakness or failure. She may not know that she needs help or know that help is available.

- Bring her interests into the curriculum. You will see her true ability and potential when you have her full engagement with a topic. Be creative – many interests can be encompassed in many subjects:

  ◦ counting Pokémon™

  ◦ English language essays based on cats

  ◦ horse care in the 19th century.

- If teamwork is necessary, give her a role that she can succeed in. Don't let her have to try to negotiate with others (social skills) to find her place. Do this with all the students if you don't want to single her out. Let them all be successful in areas where their strengths lie. She is likely to excel in planning, research and possibly writing up results.

- Reduce homework assignments. She is exhausted.

Chapter 7

Discovering Autism as an Adult

*Being different, in whatever way, seems to upset other people.
It can make them nervous, angry, abusive and indifferent, and
these reactions to me were always strong.*

LAWSON (1998, P.57)

Many of the women questioned had received their diagnosis of autism after their teenage years, some not until much later. Some of these women had spent the vast majority of their lives not knowing that they were on the autism spectrum, and having no self-awareness and no support. They grew up in a time when only children (and only male ones at that) had autism; they had to find their own way, often experiencing major crises and challenges along the way. As they were in this unique position of having experience of life both with and without diagnosis, and also with the benefit of age, I was interested to know how they felt about being autistic and being diagnosed, whether they wished that they didn't have it (if that was something they could even imagine) and whether they would have liked to have been diagnosed earlier. Their perceptions can give us insight into how girls with autism may feel in later life and help us to develop appropriate approaches to maximise the positive and minimise the negative elements of these older women's journeys. Rudy Simone asks whether Asperger Syndrome is a disability or a gift and concludes that:

> [If] you remove the autism, you remove the gifts. (Simone 2010, p.212)

She also reports on the paradox of the variable profile of challenges and abilities with an insider's insight that I think many women with autism will recognise.

> We can read books and understand anything written better than most, but can't follow social conversation. We can dismantle computers and install hardware, but can't find our way around a supermarket. We can monologue for hours on our special interests, but can't spend an hour in conversation without getting a migraine or having a meltdown. We can paint pictures and design things of astonishing beauty, but can't be bothered to fix our own hair. (Simone 2010, p.211)

The sense of difference that many women feel, I believe, stems from this uneven profile. It makes it very hard to work out where you belong when you are brilliant at things that others find hard, but useless at things that others find easy. This is why the diagnosis, at any age, can come as such a relief. It explains everything. It makes sense of everything. And women with autism need to make sense of everything.

> My head had been spinning all my life with trying to make sense of why these things happened to me, why I was so odd, why I couldn't live like other people. The diagnosis stopped my head from spinning. I was able to breathe a sigh of relief and relax. (Woman with autism)

Adult diagnosis – why bother?

One of the most common things I am asked when discussing diagnosis for adults with autism is: 'What's the point?' The presumption is that if you have made it to 40 or 50 years of age without a diagnosis and survived, why bother getting one now? My personal and professional experience paints a different picture, which is almost universal for both men and women. As one woman puts it:

> It put many of the difficulties I had with school and friendships into perspective, as well as allowing me to work out why I find some situations very stressful/tiring (e.g., social occasions, meeting new

people, loud environments etc). [...] In short, it was a massive relief – I know who I am, how I can expect myself to be, that there's nothing 'wrong' with me, and that the friendship difficulties I had weren't my fault. (Woman with autism, diagnosed aged 21 years)

What difference does diagnosis make?

Women receiving late diagnosis often share the same sense of relief and self-acceptance as men, but perhaps to an even greater degree, due to the way in which they have needed to manage their autism – often through bending to fit what's expected of them (which men with autism are seen as less prone and/or able to do). Feeling justified or vindicated by diagnosis is the strong response of many of the women I have spoken to: a sense of having the right to be yourself established – for the first time – in a world that doesn't always welcome or appreciate that self. These are women who are exhausted and angry at having tried so hard to make everything make sense, while presuming that they were to blame for not getting it in the first place; women who feel they have had to put on a persona of social acceptability in order to be tolerated. I often see individuals go through a phase of what I call 'militant' autism following diagnosis, where the person decides to behave exactly as they please, almost as a knee-jerk response to rejecting their former existence. For most people, this is part of the post-diagnostic process of coming to terms with what this new information means, and a more moderate position on how to exist more happily is usually found over time. When asked what difference having an adult diagnosis meant for them, common themes are self-acceptance and being kinder to oneself.

I have plans that are based on who I am, rather than who I think I ought to be. I spent my first half century trying to fit in and now I have stopped. If anyone questions my oddness, I tell them it's because I'm odd. (National Autistic Society 2013a)

A massive difference, mainly in terms of understanding myself and not being so hard on myself. It explained so much of my life, my needs, my choices, and it made me feel justified and validated in being how I am. It makes it easier to meet people and take on new experiences because I know why I find things difficult, I know what might help, and if it doesn't work I am more accepting. It helps with the guilt – why didn't I travel the world during my gap year, why aren't I using my PhD to commute to London to work a 50-hour-a-week job, why don't I go to parties when I am invited, why do I not enjoy parties I do go to when I have guilted myself into going, etc. (Woman with autism, diagnosed aged 31 years)

[The diagnosis] wasn't unexpected but the emotions that came afterwards were. I feel I am in a period of 'mourning'; not sure how I feel about it and what it means. (Woman with autism, recently diagnosed aged 48 years)

Before the diagnosis I'd thought I had no friends because I was unpleasant; then I learned that it was simply difficult for me to communicate in the way that makes people comfortable forming bonds of friendship. Before the diagnosis, when I 'withdrew' it had always been attributed to me being 'moody' or 'sulky', when actually, inside, I often felt calm and happy and was surprised when people were angry. It explained why I had difficulty functioning in a typical way and found day-to-day life such a challenge. (Woman with autism, diagnosed aged 33 years)

For the most part, people reflect my own attitude – it's not a big deal, it's just who I am, and for those who knew me before the diagnosis, it's obvious I'm still the same person. It's as much a part of me as the colour of my hair or my love of music; it's just not as visible in the same way. My ex-fiancé's reaction wasn't as positive – he expressed a concern that our children would have autism, and accused me of using it as a 'crutch' to 'excuse' behaviours that he didn't find acceptable. (Woman with autism, diagnosed aged 21 years)

Do you wish you didn't have autism?
This is a big question to ask and a hard one to answer (we're not supposed to be good at imagining what it's like to be someone else).

I was interested to know if the fact of having made it to adulthood – as a person with autism in a neurotypical (NT) governed world – had given them a sense that being one of those NTs would have been preferable. For most – perhaps surprisingly, considering the difficult lives they had often had – this was not the case. Their comments and insights were considered, sometimes militantly proud, sometimes sad, sometimes angry, acknowledging regrets and missed opportunities. Some recognised and were happy with who they were in themselves as people, but frustrated and tired by the negative consequences that they had experienced in their lives at the hands of an NT world that did not understand and accept their way of being.

> Yes, it would have been easier through the years. So many situations in life have been difficult to navigate. (Woman with autism)

> Sometimes I wish that I didn't have autism, but mostly because of the anxiety side of things. (Woman with autism)

> I wish it was accepted and that I didn't have such a lonely life. (Woman with autism)

> I'd have to know what life was like as an NT to make that decision. I would prefer not to have the sensory issues but the heightened memory and 'cutting through the bullshit' aspects of the condition are actually mildly appealing as character traits. I *almost* wish more people were definitively on the spectrum to make 'us' the majority in society. (Woman with autism)

> Yes […] and no in some respects. Since receiving the diagnosis I have gained a slightly better appreciation of myself, and pride myself in finding worth in my various personality niggles. I do loathe how difficult it is for me to engage in typical discourse, and also my panic attacks when it comes to confronting the big, wide, human world. It's those public inhibitions where I want to express myself or get my point across that do bother me at times, but I am glad for what I know about my (though maybe limited to some) interests. (Woman with autism)

Mostly the women felt happy to be autistic and had no desire to be different, despite the challenges they had faced. It must be noted that the type of person who willingly contributes to autism research such as this is more likely to be someone who is aware and knowledgeable about their condition and perhaps is more likely to feel positive about it than someone less educated about it. In my experience of working with young women with autism, this positivity is not always so evident at an earlier age. When younger, the desire to fit in is enormous, as we have heard. Age, and with it self-acceptance, appears to play a big part in feeling OK about your autism. In some of the women, pride in their identity and, dare I say it, contempt for NT values are evident.

> No, because then I wouldn't be me. You don't take off the autistic part and discover a 'normal' person underneath. I am autistic the way you have blue eyes or curly hair. It goes all the way through, like letters in seaside rock. It governs the way I think, listen to my body, the way my body talks back to me, how I see the world, everything. (Woman with autism)

> I am glad that I have autism, I find the NTs confusing, like sheep following each other around. They never seem to say what they mean. I try to avoid them. (Woman with autism)

> I am proud to be autistic. Do you ever look objectively at NTs? Yes, some are good, but many routinely tell lies, exclude those who are different, subscribe to superficial trends, talk nonsense and are obsessed with conformity. Why would I want to be NT? Ugh. (Woman with autism)

> Autism makes me very unique, and in principle I don't mind being different. I know I am very capable and very intelligent in a unique way. I just wish I had the social skills to be able to do something good with that set of skills. (Woman with autism)

Would you have liked to have been diagnosed earlier?

Current thinking suggests that early diagnosis, and therefore appropriate support and intervention, is in the best interests of individuals with autism. The women questioned had varying responses, with the majority feeling that an earlier diagnosis could have given them access to opportunities that had been denied to them due to an inability to access support; they also felt it could have saved them from a lot of emotional pain and the feeling that there was something very wrong with them. Interestingly, several women said they would have liked to have been diagnosed earlier than they were, but not necessarily in childhood. They felt that a childhood diagnosis may have resulted in limitations placed on them by themselves and also by others in their lives: parents and teachers, who may have tried to protect them.

> I would definitely have liked to have been diagnosed earlier. I spent the first 13 years of my life thinking I was nothing but a freak (that mindset still sticks with me today), simply because that's how the world viewed me. (Woman with autism)

> I feel I have sacrificed the gifts from my Aspieness in order to fit in. Maybe if I had been diagnosed earlier I would not have spent a whole life trying to fit in, and would have been able to forgive my own social deficits, thus saving the energy and intellect required to pretend to be normal, which I could have dedicated to things that I really wanted to do, such as research into science and/or languages. (Woman with autism)

> It would've changed my entire life, in short. It wouldn't have allowed my chronic depression, which coincided with my not knowing what was 'wrong' with me during that crucial time of my life, to overwhelm me or leave me awash with the cycle of perpetual procrastination that it did. It condemned me to an abyss of endless inaction. I still resent those more professional people around me for not spotting the signs sooner. (Woman with autism)

The women who commented that they would not have wanted an earlier diagnosis felt that they were stronger and more capable because of what they had been through. Some of them felt that children diagnosed nowadays are sometimes overprotected and, as a result, are less independent than they were.

> Positives would have been maybe getting some help, support and understanding. Negatives would have been having my aspirations downgraded – you can't manage that, it would be too stressful etc., and seeing yourself as less and defective. (Woman with autism)

> [Maybe] but any early intervention/help may ultimately have hindered my development into the adult I've become – I believe I'm stronger through having struggled at times and am far more prepared for the nature of adult life than some people who have had support for years. (Woman with autism)

> I probably wouldn't have been nearly so independent and self-reliant as I am today […] When I see so many young people with Asperger's who seem to be so protected (by their mums especially), I don't think it's good for them. I think the parents don't realise how much their son or daughter could do if they were encouraged more instead of being made to feel they are disabled. (Woman with autism)

Chapter 8

You Don't Look Autistic

*There are times when I am in 'professional' mode and the
person I am with would probably never believe I was autistic.
They might think I am younger than I am or a little eccentric
but otherwise perfectly 'normal'.*

LAWSON (1998, P.111)

Adult characteristics and looking 'normal'

As adolescence passes and adulthood ensues, expectations and
requirements change, but autism remains. With research and support
firmly focused on children with autism, adults plough on regardless.
For our women, many of whom have spent their childhood and teenage
years learning how to mask their difficulties hide and slip under the
radar of weirdness, adulthood is merely a continuation of that facade
along with a whole set of new and increased requirements to be
independent, navigate the adult world and perhaps earn a wage.

From the reports of women who contributed to my survey, my own
professional personal experiences and those of other authors, one
thing is patently clear: women with autism are a lot more 'autistic' than
they look.

All of the diagnostic criteria for autism remain for these women, but
are simply presented differently as an adult. Professionals must take
into account what a lifetime of autistic experience can result in when
assessing and working with adults. Of course we don't 'look' the same
as a child with autism. No adult is the same as they were as a child,
regardless of the presence of autism.

The majority of these women are getting through each day with an often sophisticated set of compensatory behaviours, personas and clever strategies for avoiding certain situations without anyone knowing. Their ability to do this is testament to an extraordinary resilience and sometimes stubborn determination not to 'fail' or be 'outed' as a 'weirdo'. Unfortunately, these efforts can come at a price: exhaustion, breakdown and other mental health issues are commonly mentioned by these women. These ill-effects are the consequences of living with autism, not conditions or symptoms to be considered in isolation. This is an important point that clinicians must address. Life with autism can break a person. The symptoms of the breakage are not the issues to be treated or addressed; the difficulty of living in a neurotypical (NT) world with autism is the key. We will look at health implications in Chapter 13. This chapter will focus on the core characteristics of autism that adult women report as having an impact on their lives. Headings will differ from those in the chapters about children as many childhood issues become less evident or important. For example, while adult women still find eye contact and facial expressions difficult to interpret, they understand that these are important, so may use them mechanically by rote, even if not intuitively, resulting in what appears to be NT behaviour.

> As years go by, you get better and better at camouflaging and compensating for the external behavioural characteristics of autism. You make the impression of functioning normally by cognitively compensating for what you do not sense or know intuitively due to your autistic way of thinking. (Jansen and Rombout 2014, p.23)

I wanted to know what benefits and skills the women felt they gained from having autism (we must not forget that this profile has both its advantages and disadvantages). In order to live well with autism I believe it is necessary to gain self-acceptance and self-esteem, which requires the person to appreciate and embrace who they are. Traits that the women liked in themselves were focused on their determination and ability to challenge themselves in difficult times. As shown by the examples below, many women did have positive feelings about themselves, almost in spite of their negative experiences at the hands of an NT world.

> Being independent, learning to cope with adversity, being determined when I want to learn something new, being good at trying things such as DIY so I have become quite good at it. I am very arty and possibly having AS [Asperger Syndrome] has helped with that. I am honest, too, and caring and thoughtful. (Woman with autism)

> I love my sense of duty, my sense of rightness and justice, and my honesty. I will return change to a shop because it is WRONG to keep it if it isn't mine. My passion for reading means I have specialist knowledge on very niche subjects, and I enjoy that. (Woman with autism)

> Ability to become immersed in secondary (fantasy) worlds. Sense of the ridiculous and unusual humour (probably seen sometimes by others as childishness). Understanding and communication with animals and appreciation of the natural world. Having an analytical mind. Intense focus and attention to detail. Being different and being unique. Sense of morality and opposition to injustice. Being trustworthy and dependable. (Woman with autism)

Characteristics

When considering the characteristics of autism that manifest most significantly for these adult women, we must continue to bear in mind societal expectations for women. For example, you will read quotes from women below who hate to share their things; this is not acceptable behaviour for an adult woman who is supposed to be sharing and caring. While some of these characteristics may be equally applicable to men with autism, the gender expectation factor may increase the negative response to these traits from others (which therefore increases the impact on self-esteem and consequently mental health).

Non-verbal characteristics

As mentioned above, adult women with autism have often learned that facial expressions, body language and eye contact are required if one wishes to fit into the NT world without remonstration, and they have become rather good at presenting themselves in a manner that does not attract attention. They are often keenly aware of how they have constructed a means of minimising discomfort while maximising invisibility and social inclusion. These women start out as 'little psychologists' and by adulthood can be masters at analysing social behaviour and emulating it. It must be noted that this is usually not intuitive; it involves conscious awareness and effort 100 per cent of the time while in any social environment, which is draining.

> I do eye contact, but I'm a mouth reader. Eye contact is completely distracting for me although I have learned that if you look in between the eyes, the other person will think you are doing the whole eyeball thing. (Woman with autism)

Even those who do not find masking their differences easy show an incredible awareness of what they 'get wrong' and how they compensate, despite having no means (and in some cases, no desire) of fixing it and doing otherwise.

> Intense eye contact once obtained (staring sternly), rated people's intent purely on the basis of voice, being capable of understanding only the most apparent facial expressions (but would have trouble telling if say, a smile was a genuine smile and not just a strained one even then). I still rely on intonation to tell me what I need to know about a person's emotions. (Woman with autism)

> As an adult, people often ask if I am OK. I really don't know what my face is saying. (Woman with autism)

This last comment reminds me of a situation where I was being photographed for a magazine article. I thought I was giving the photographer my best smile, but then he said, 'You look like you want to kill me'. This was a major revelation at the age of 42 when I realised that what I thought I was expressing on my face was nothing like the reality. It explained why 'smile, it might never happen' has been a common and, up until now, bemusing, comment from complete strangers throughout my life. This prompted me to spend several hours looking in a mirror and I realised that my face doesn't move anywhere near as much as I thought it did.

Communication skills

Diagnostically, the ability to participate in two-way conversation is a core part of the Autism Spectrum Disorder (ASD) criteria. Women with autism tend to be direct, straightforward and blunt in their communication style due to difficulties picking up the subtleties of non-verbal cues. These are not typically 'female' traits and are often received very negatively. The woman herself is often bemused as to why she has caused such a response, since from her perspective she was only stating the truth or asking directly for the clarity she needed. In Chapter 6, it was suggested that girls with autism are treated less favourably than boys when it comes to perceived rudeness, and this does not abate in adulthood. With regard to small talk, adult women with ASD don't like it or 'get it' any more than they did when they were teenagers. Difficulties with non-verbal cues can also result in interrupting and missing the flow of conversation. This, combined with a preference for talking about oneself and one's own interests, all add up to someone whose conversation style is not always appreciated. The specific impacts of this communication profile on friendships and relationships are discussed in Chapters 9 and 11.

> I've been told I'm very blunt and direct, and I often offend people without meaning to. Apparently I come across as aggressive. I like to get to the point of something, and all the superfluous detail irritates me. (Woman with autism)

> I still have issues with turn-taking in conversation. If I don't say something the second I think of it, then it is lost – often forever – so I interrupt a lot and talk over people. I'd say I'm more aware of when

I'm interrupting than I used to be and better at reining myself in when necessary. (Woman with autism)

I can be very self-centred. These days I have to make a conscious effort to pretend to be interested in how somebody else is so I can be considered nice, but really all I want to do is talk about myself. (Woman with autism)

The result of these communication differences can be that women with autism misunderstand the words of others as well as being misunderstood themselves. Jokes, sarcasm and a tendency to take things literally can cause confusion, anxiety and a general feeling of stupidity at not having 'got it'. This is not to say that women with autism do not have a sense of humour, and they may be quick-witted with their own jokes; but the jokes of others may be lost on them at times. I have been told on more than one occasion that I can't have autism because I have a sense of humour and know how to tell a joke. While this is true, I am still unable to tell if someone else is joking, will believe pretty much anything I am told, and yet refuse to believe something that has been said is a joke when I'm told that it is. Something that often comes up in my conversations with women with autism about the causes of their frustrations is why people say they will do something and then don't do it or do something else. The discrepancy between people's words and actions is not only stressful due to the change in expectations that has to be processed (hard work), but also because it is not true and therefore illogical. There is nothing that stresses a person with autism more than a lack of logic or an unnecessary lie – we find it baffling. The unanswerable question of autism, which is always accompanied by a creased forehead, is: 'Why do people do that?' I once (jokingly) said at a conference that I wanted the forehead crease so often seen in women with autism to be called 'Hendrickx Syndrome'. This talk was filmed and put onto YouTube. Since then, so many women have contacted me to tell me that this is also true of them that perhaps I should pursue this route to infamy. My partner is constantly smoothing out the crease on my forehead. He says I have two facial expressions: puzzled and surprised.

Having their own words and motivations so frequently misunderstood leads women with autism to self-censorship, requiring them to be on 'red alert' to every single thought before they utter it. Even with this filter in place, social faux pas are common because the filter itself does not know what to look for. I find all conversation fraught with anxiety as I anticipate that at any given second, I might say something that will offend, confuse or alert my audience to my lack of fluency in my native social language. This fear is not Social Anxiety Disorder in the sense that it is irrational and psychological in origin. The fear is based on evidence and fact and is wholly rational: it happens frequently and is due to a lack of cognitive skills in this area.

Sharing

As discussed in Chapter 4, in early childhood females with autism have difficulties with the concept of sharing, and for some that doesn't go away. They may have learned that sharing is something that is required and will concede without complaint, but that does not mean that it comes easily. Lending or sharing an item means a loss of control and not knowing where that item is, along with a feeling of insecurity: 'How will I get it back?' This is associated with a preference for routine, sameness and a dislike of change – specifically, change that is implemented by others. All of these elements encompass the same basic stressors: 'I don't know how to make sense of this and how to maintain control'. Controlling possessions, tasks and environments reduces stress and anxiety. Women with autism are generally not team-players and prefer to go it alone when doing tasks and projects.

The sharing of space when co-habiting causes issues. One of the key factors in my own ability to function well is knowing where every single item I possess is – always. I never need to worry about not having what I need or having to look for it. I know where to find what I will require at any given moment in time; therefore stress is reduced to zero. Living with other people means that things are moved. The impact of this is huge for me – far greater than simply the annoyance of having to look for or ask for something. The certainty of my personal physical world is the foundation of my existence, and it is hard for others to understand that my extreme distress at someone having moved the sticky tape is not an over-reaction or a sign of mental illness; it's all an easily explainable part of my autism.

> Very leery of lending people anything, even in the event of loaning something as meagre or trivial as a pencil. Far too aware of the time that each person spent with a loaned item as well, and would be combative if someone was notably 'hogging' something for long periods when compared with the rest of those concerned. (Woman with autism)

> I do not share. Over the years, for the few times I have shared, I have learned that I will never get whatever I shared back in any form, nor will the kindness be reciprocated at any point in time. (Woman with autism)

> I hate people to be in my space and my stuff [...] When I moved in with my husband I completely freaked out for at least a year. He is now well and truly part of the furniture! (Woman with autism)

Sensory behaviours

Obvious and visible repetitive motor mannerisms are usually more associated with individuals with autism who have an intellectual disability, but the adult women I questioned, none of whom had any learning disability, mentioned finding certain movements and behaviours either enjoyable or increasing at times of stress. By far the most common was finger picking. As a fellow finger-picker, I can say that I am largely unaware of doing this beyond the small and disgusting piles of skin that I leave behind. For me, there is a need for constant movement even when sitting still, along with an urge for perfection – if I feel a rough edge to my skin around my fingers I have to try to get rid of it. This (obviously) tends not to work and creates more uneven skin. This usually results in sore and bleeding fingers. There is a tic/Tourette Syndrome-type automatic response at work here for me, and perhaps this is the case for others, given that co-morbidity of other neurodiverse conditions alongside the autism is to be expected. This should not be mistaken for Obsessive Compulsive Disorder, which involves a different cognitive process.

Scratching, picking, rubbing and plucking hairs all featured as typical sensory behaviours. Many of these are not regarded as particularly unusual per se, but it is their intensity and frequency that demonstrate a difference. It is also the case that this type of behaviour is often attributed to anxiety disorders, but while this may be the case for women with autism, it also may not be. Individuals with autism are known to find solace and relaxation in repetitive movements and therefore it should not automatically be assumed that behaviours of this type are a problem or only arise during anxiety. I find that picking and hair-pulling put me into a trance-like, almost meditative state, which is deeply relaxing and all-consuming. I have no desire to stop these behaviours and can manage them so that they do not cause me any physical harm. Understanding the function of the behaviour to the individual is necessary before suggesting it stops. Cessation without meeting that core need in some other less harmful way may provoke the inception of a new and more harmful physical response.

I really, really enjoy spinning. I have a special spinny chair so that I can spin at home. (Woman with autism)

I have found that, especially more recently as my life has been getting so much more stressful, I am stimming a lot, usually scratching myself, particularly my arms. To counteract this, I have acquired a bracelet which I am using as a stimming bracelet. (Woman with autism)

Tap foot or pat knee. Press foot down to ground, flex arm tense so much to cause bruise on arm, squeeze jaw with cheeks pressed in, clench teeth, hold steering wheel very firmly. (Woman with autism)

At times of stress I've found that plucking hairs out of my legs is very therapeutic. I don't think this is really self-harming; it only hurts a bit. (Woman with autism)

The sensory tolerance differences in individuals with autism are well reported. Most of the women I questioned did not report significant difficulties in accessing the world due to specific sensory sensitivities. The most commonly mentioned issues were crowded places and situations that were overwhelming from a holistic sensory perspective, rather than because of one particular sensory stressor. Heightened sensory responses were not always perceived as negative – many women with autism report a wonderful intensity of sensation and attention to stimuli that those without autism do not have, and this brings them huge pleasure. Feeling particularly in tune with visual beauty and nature was a common theme.

> I usually have some soft material in a pocket that I can run my fingers over to gain reassurance. Occasionally, I enjoy sitting in the bedroom cupboard, closing off from all outside disturbances. (Lawson 1998, p.102)

> I have major problems with light […] I do not like unexpected touch and will flinch, push away or go rigid when others touch me […] Smells make me retch, quiet noises like leaves rustling or birds tweeting engulf my brain. However, I do feel blessed because although the unpleasant stuff is heightened, so is the good stuff. Certain music makes my brain dance […] I feel very attached and deeply moved by the beauty of nature too. (Woman with autism)

Coping with change and uncertainty

Surprisingly, given the often independent and high-functioning lives (as parents, academics and employees) that the women participants lead, their struggles with changes of plans and breaks to routines are significant. You would often never know that these women are finding things so tough. Their tendency is to tell the world that this new situation is fine, take the stress on themselves and do what is required, but then go home and cry and/or engage in self-destructive behaviours. I hate it when people change plans, but I never let it show because I'm supposed to be flexible. This leads people to think that I can handle anything. I tell them it's fine, but it's not fine. It's never fine. When they have gone my head hurts with the effort of making sense of why they couldn't do what they said they were going to do, what it will mean for me to have to reconfigure everything to take into account the new situation and what bad things I can wish upon them for being so unreliable.

Mental health conditions are the outcome of this refusal to admit limitations. Admission of limitations equates to failure for many women with autism. Admitting vulnerability and asking for concessions or help is hard after a lifetime of masking.

> I get physical feelings of anxiety. I have learned to hold it in when in the workplace, although not always successfully, and have spent many a lunch hour hiding in the work toilets hyperventilating and sobbing uncontrollably. I used to feel pathetic when this happened; I now realise since diagnosis how incredibly brave I was, actually pulling myself together and going back to work for the afternoon, before collapsing through my front door when I got home, feeling such distress and anxiety. (Woman with autism)

> Dislike of changes to plans or vague plans when trying to plan outfit/ shoes/things appropriate to activity/location/weather – intense dislike of feeling wrongly dressed or not having the right things with me. (Woman with autism)

> Changes, even minor ones, to routines upset me greatly and cause my behaviour to become challenging [...] A few weeks ago I had a meltdown because my mum was home half an hour late from walking the dog and I had planned to do something at that time, and losing that half hour threw me out of my routine and ruined my whole day. She bore the brunt of my anger; it's a good thing she loves me unconditionally. (Woman with autism)

Like the girls with autism, the women maintain routines and schedules that ensure a level of certainty and predictability in their lives. These things provide structure and limit stress and anxiety. They should not be seen as a problem unless they are so restrictive that they are detrimental to a woman living her life and her ability to function. Many women adhere to a number of routines and procedures throughout their day, but these will not be immediately obvious and may be deliberately hidden. I will not answer the door or the phone if I don't know who it is. I am seen as a very able and independent person, but I suffer extreme anxiety at the prospect of leaving the house, even to go to the local shop. I have developed strategies to hide this from other people. It is surprisingly easy to maintain a required structure without anyone being aware that I am enabling my own need for predictable outcomes. The majority of NT individuals are not terribly observant when it comes to recognising that someone in the office always wears the same clothes every Tuesday or drinks their tea from a specific mug. Maintaining these small measures may make the difference between a woman with autism feeling secure and able to cope with her day or feeling completely overwhelmed and ineffective because her markers of certainty have been lost.

> My whole life revolves around routines [...] I go through phases of obsessiveness, so I might eat the same food over and over again for weeks and then change. I get stuck on a song and replay it over and over again. These issues have always been the same throughout my life. I don't see it as a problem. (Woman with autism)

Fantasy worlds and imaginary friends

The fantasy world described in the childhood experiences of girls with autism still exists for a number of adult women, and why wouldn't it? The escape from a difficult world that imaginary worlds offered her childhood self is needed just as much in adult life. The processing and running through of events and scenarios may be a useful strategy for making sense of situations and providing respite from a life that does not offer the emotional highs and predictability of the literature that many of these girls and women have been reading voraciously since childhood. Real life is dull and scary by comparison. Unless there is a genuine concern that the person cannot determine fantasy from reality and is in danger of harm, I would argue that these worlds and characters play a valuable role for women with autism in coping with life and should be accepted for what they are.

> I currently only have one imaginary friend, who takes the form of my late best friend/love. He often works as my common sense when I'm deep in anxiety, reassuring me that the things I think are just warped perceptions. I will often talk to him out loud. (Woman with autism)

> Fantasise about living in a different part of the country and starting over, kind of like witness protection, cutting all ties to my present life […] like a new identity. (Woman with autism)

> I assumed the persona of many an alternate being when feeling overwhelmed or threatened. My perception of my surroundings would be engulfed by the sensations I imagined my 'other me' would experience. It was essentially an alternate universe. This fantasy world persists to this day, and my need to re-imagine the mundane. (Woman with autism)

> I never had imaginary friends, but [from] a teenager onwards I did have imaginary lovers. I dreamed up plenty [of] imaginary worlds. I love fantasy literature and that has continued to fuel those imaginary worlds. (Woman with autism)

Clothes

Something I noted in the girls with autism was their choice of clothing, which was selected for function rather than fashion. For many of the women questioned, this remains the case. Unless fashion is a specific interest or passion, it is largely irrelevant to the majority of women with autism I have met. Some women described an androgynous appearance and choice of clothing; others had strong preferences for certain colours, textures or styles. Plain, in general, was preferred to anything overly ornate or fussy; and if something fits and works, buying a number of the same item (possibly in different colours if she is feeling particularly frivolous) makes logical sense. Shoes, handbags, jewellery and other accessories are not something that I see on most of the women with autism that I meet. I spend the vast majority of my life in two sets of footwear: boots for winter and flip-flops for summer. I have more recently come to realise that wearing dresses avoids the stress involved in finding two items (or more) that match. This gives me the appearance of being fashion-conscious, feminine and thus more invisible. My dresses are all cotton, stretchy and have stripes. Stripes are the only way I can wear more than one colour without fear of choosing a pattern that the rest of the world has decreed to be revolting or tasteless, while I remain oblivious. I have no idea why one flowery dress is considered nice while another may be deemed awful. Flowers are flowers to me; I have no means of discerning current trends. I have no major interest in fashion, but I do not wish to be viewed negatively and so conforming (usually) ensures anonymity. If a friend asks what I think about her new handbag, I find myself unable to speak; despite trawling through my brain for something, anything, to say, I cannot muster a single word as I have absolutely no opinion on handbags beyond it's a bag, it carries stuff.

> My clothes are very samey and simple [...] My husband thinks I am hilarious and brilliant at the same time. I am in and out of the shops in a flash. My new winter coat this year was virtually identical to last year's; he laughed so much when he saw it. (Woman with autism)

> I tend to wear simple clothing that could just as easily be worn by a man (albeit a small one). Of course I am aware of gender expectations and will wear high heels if the occasion requires it, although I think that even when I dress feminine, my style is always a little bit manly. (Woman with autism)

Interests

As life gets in the way of the all-encompassing pursuit of passions and intense interests, these get side-lined by the need for domestic and occupational obligations, but they still exist. (Musicians/bands, TV shows, science fiction and video-gaming were all favourite interests among the women I questioned.) Reading and gathering knowledge about special interests (often carried over from childhood) was still a huge draw for these women. The intensity of interest is still as great as it is for males, but the form of the interest can differ. Rather than simply focusing on the story being told, it is the people in TV shows and movies that can become obsessions, as both the character and the actor themselves. However, the topics of the shows are often science fiction – in line with typical male interests. Many interests enjoyed by women with autism can appear as fairly common – soap operas, cooking, travel – but, again, the depth of knowledge and the diligence put into the learning is way in excess of a 'hobby'. I am obsessed with living as naturally as possible. I try to cook as much of my own food as I can, including baking bread, making ice cream and all my own juices. This sounds like something that many people do, but for me it is more fulfilling than that. If I have to buy a loaf of bread, I feel physically sick and agitated because I have not made it myself. If I pick fruit from a tree, I feel intense emotions and joy.

> I have got into debt before in pursuit of my collecting. I set myself a weekly Amazon budget now (I will do without clothes/toiletries to buy my books) for my books to control this. The book thing has always been a special interest of mine […] It's not just about the content of the book for me; I actually like the book itself. I only like paperbacks because I like to feel the smooth, cool embossed covers and I like to flick the pages. I like the way a book smells and looks when [it is] on a bookshelf. (Woman with autism)

> Over the years I have bought a whole load of musical instruments. I can't play any of them. I have tried but I have no prowess or talent for music. I am so in awe of people who can play together harmoniously in a group. It makes me cry with intense emotion. It seems like magic. The instruments themselves are so beautifully crafted. I feel enormous joy just to hold them.' (Woman with autism)

Sleep

Sleep was mentioned as a problem for some women I interviewed. The 'buzzy' head mentioned by younger girls seems to persist for some older women. The need to 'file' and process the day that has passed and to anticipate the one to come appears to prevent easy rest. Difficulty in getting to sleep was most commonly mentioned.

> Thinking of lots of stuff, like what happened that day, what [I'm] going to do next day. (Woman with autism)

> I describe my mind like the inside of a beehive, busy and crammed [...] If I wake in the night [...] my brain switches on and starts whirring. It drives me bonkers. (Woman with autism)

Independent skills

As mentioned previously, many women with autism manage to remain invisible and appear capable on the surface, so it is perhaps surprising to understand the extent of the challenges they face each day. A number of these challenges impact behind closed doors in the home, where personal skills, housekeeping and cooking can be shielded from the gaze of the outside world – and we know how adept these women are at hiding things.

> Housekeeping has always confounded me. I either become hyperfocused on one small aspect of a task and accomplish nothing else, or I scream in torment as I realise I have gone in circles, starting multiple tasks and finishing none. (Kearns Miller 2003, p.215)

> Getting dressed and washed is difficult for me. I get things in the wrong order or might miss something out altogether, like forgetting to wash my armpits or something. To deal with this I have very strict routines: I wash my body in exactly the same way every time [...] If I get interrupted though, it's a different matter [...] If I reached for the shampoo and the bottle wasn't where it should be, I would find it very difficult to deal with that. (Woman with autism)

Simple tasks take considerable energy and resources, leaving less for the complicated matters of dealing with people.

> I've had trouble initiating communication with strangers, the sort of situation where you ask a stranger for directions or something, I've spent a lot of time lost because I didn't want to approach a stranger. (Woman with autism)

> I have always been very sensitive to and overwhelmed by crowds and I have felt panicked and lost in a turbulent sea of people. Likewise, I was always frightened of going alone to public places and have always needed others to help me feel grounded in public locations, sometimes needing them to be my guide through chaotic types of environment. (Woman with autism)

I have worked with women who live in complete chaos at home, but who are extremely ordered at work. They feel totally overwhelmed with the ongoing and more abstract nature of tasks at home (there is no real schedule unless you impose one on yourself) and find the accountability of a regime in the workplace easier to adhere to.

Years of experience and necessity have led women to develop their own awareness and consequently to develop strategies to overcome some of their practical challenges. For some this has been the result of getting into difficulty and having to make sure that this is not repeated. Disabling the door bell in order not to have to hear it or answer it was mentioned by one woman (Jansen and Rombout 2014) as a means of having more control over her environment and reducing potential anxiety.

> I dislike answering the door phone, but will do it when necessary. I also tend to fall behind with housework and administrative stuff including bills, and I have a 'master list' to try and keep myself on track. (Woman with autism)

One lady has produced a guidance sheet for interacting with people on public transport. She had listed how many times one should smile at the driver in order to avoid 'making a fool of' oneself.

She explained that reviewing social interactions and analysing them in order to identify where things went wrong takes up a huge amount of her time and, of course, this is exhausting. (ASD Specialist Support Worker)

I manage money by making sure every single bill debits my account on payday [...] I could not cope with payments leaving my account throughout the month. I have got into financial trouble as a result. (Woman with autism)

I still struggle sometimes with things like phoning up to order a take-away; I'm very grateful that modern technology means I can order food without having to deal with a human being. (Woman with autism)

The impact of the profile of autism may lessen for some over the course of a lifetime, but this benefit is balanced by the increasing requirements placed on an adult as opposed to a child. We know that women with autism are particularly invisible in their presentation of the diagnostic characteristics, but we also know that this invisibility is a smokescreen that fails to alert us to the true extent of the challenges these women are facing every single day.

Chapter 9

Adult Relationships

Somebody asked me recently if there might not be some way in which I could enjoy doing social things. How about, he said, if we removed the pressure of expectations (to react, to talk) and kept the number of people to two or three and didn't get noisy, etc., etc. Well, I answered, if you took away all the things that make me not like socializing, I guess the answer is, yes, I might like that kind of social activity.

KEARNS MILLER (2003, P.239)

Friends and other people

We will talk about personal and sexual relationships in Chapter 11, but for now, let's talk about friends.

> Still not sure what that really means, what it takes to be a friend. (Woman with autism)

Friendships and people interactions continue to be a major source of analysis, effort and anxiety for adult women with autism. Adulthood for some brings a greater degree of self-acceptance and awareness of the types of people and interactions that work best. The trying, difficult teenage years are left behind and real choices about who to spend one's time with arise. The issues with friends are three-fold: first is the matter of identifying who might become a potential friend and knowing when they have become one; second, is the actual social effort and understanding required to physically spend time in their presence; and, third, is the understanding of how the friendship needs to be maintained (through contact) in-between meetings. All of these factors affect the ability of women with autism to make and keep friends, and to tolerate the presence of other people to ensure long-term social contact; all are also directly attributable to the core diagnostic criteria of autism.

> I see the way some of my acquaintances act towards other friends of theirs and they seem to have this [...] give-and-take/back-and-forth, sort of interaction which looks totally effortless. (Woman with autism)

The issue of friends is a complex one throughout life for these women with Autism Spectrum Disorder (ASD) and it takes many years to get their heads around either what it means to be a friend or how to be around people without anxiety and fear of rejection and social failure. All those years of childhood feelings of difference take their toll and leave their mark.

> I am beginning to discover what it is like to enjoy the company of someone else and not feel afraid. (Lawson 1998, p.12)

Personally, I have about five people that I spend any time with outside my immediate family (partner and children). They are either men or women diagnosed with autism, those with considerable autistic traits, or gay men. I do not have any neurotypical (NT) female or straight male friends; these two groups are too socially complicated and frightening for me to cope with (gay men are safer because the potential misread/missed attraction issue is removed). I see each of these people individually on average at three-month intervals, although sometimes much longer apart. It is quite usual for me not to see anyone apart from my partner for several months at a time. I make virtually no contact with these people unless it is to arrange a meeting or discuss a specific point or question. I do not miss their company and would probably not notice much if I never saw any of them again, even though I really like them and care about their well-being. The number of people I have felt a genuine 'rapport' with during my life is in single figures. The number of people who have ever witnessed my entire 'real' self is one. Experience has taught me that generally it is not safe to reveal all.

My world is extremely self-centric and focused on my projects, plans and existence. It simply wouldn't occur to me to invite a friend for a walk or a bike ride, for example; I would just go by myself. I like these people very much, but find that after around two hours I have run out of things to say, have exhausted myself with 'performing' and need to leave, go home and have a nap. Even when I look relaxed, the constant awareness that things could go wrong at any second never leaves me. I watch groups of people having what looks like fun together and feel intense sadness at not ever having experienced such ease around people and the natural acceptance of each other's quirks that they seem to have. Paradoxically, I find most people extremely irritating, facile and socially dishonest, which means that the likelihood of me ever finding my 'gang' is pretty small! From my discussions with other women with autism, I would suggest that my experiences are not atypical. The frequency of interactions and number of people in the women's lives were typically small. They tended to meet on a one-to-one and fairly intermittent basis. For most, this was enough to meet their social requirements. For one woman, her partner was the only person she needed in her life. The quality of their relationship provided her with what most women with autism are looking for: acceptance without judgement.

> I never meet up with friends and have no desire to. My best friend is my husband; he truly accepts me for me. He has held my hand without judgement for the last ten years and I love him so much. (Woman with autism)

Interactions were reported to be exhausting, requiring both preparation and post-meeting respite. Women describe their awareness of personas and scripts to help get them through essential interactions with the outside world.

> Every social encounter requires constant decoding and then selection of an appropriate response. I have preprogrammed/ learned behaviours for church, meals, restaurants, casual, semi-casual, formal situations. (Kearns Miller 2003, p.255)

> I feel as if I've restarted my life many times, even taking on a new persona in each phase of my life. I can cut myself off from events in my past to the extent that they feel like they happened to someone else. (Woman with autism)

What we can learn from these women is that large social networks are not the norm and that crafting a social world that fits within the autism is the best path to well-being. If women with autism can understand that their 'failure' to procure a large group of friends is actually perfectly typical, I hope this will lead to a greater sense of self-worth and acceptance.

> For me, even interacting with friends I've known for years is difficult. I have to make a conscious effort to sort of 'keep on task' when I am with a friend. So in the end, I am exhausted, and just can't face seeing them again anytime soon. (Woman with autism)

> I would say there are only three people I see once every few months, and I consider them to be my friends. Yet, even with them I feel like now somewhat we have not much to say to each other. (Woman with autism)

> My best friend lives in New York and I usually see her [a] couple of times a year and chat to her on the phone or online/text about once a week. Recently, she's been visiting more often and this has been a bit of a problem. I don't know how to tell her I don't want to see her so much without offending her but I find her visits very tiring. (Woman with autism)

For some there was a sense that seeing other people 'got in the way' of them doing their own preferred activities. This, I would argue, is in direct contrast to most NT women who would choose socialising and companionship over solo pursuits.

> I have some other friends who I see occasionally, perhaps once every two months. This suits me fine as I find people hard work and I simply don't have the time and energy to spend it socialising when there's other things I need to do. (Woman with autism)

For some of the women, their social interactions had to have some purpose or function; the idea of simply meeting others to chat held no appeal. It is commonly considered that sharing interests is a core facet of autistic relationships, and these women are no different in that respect. There was a sense of the relationship being on their terms and needing to meet their requirements, rather than for the purpose of establishing a mutual, empathic and emotional bond, in most cases.

> I don't want more friends really. That would be too much to take on […] I suppose ideally I'd like a friend who was knowledgeable about IT and would give me free IT help, but that is the only addition I would consider making. (Woman with autism)

> I can be a 'user' in friendships, I like people who know more about things than I do, so I make an effort to befriend people who are clever and know things. I have a very low tolerance for people I perceive as stupid. (Woman with autism)

> My friendships are more based on a mutual exchange of knowledge and/or practical help or advice. We don't do 'small talk' or meet for a coffee for no apparent reason. All interactions have a purpose. I suppose some might say we're just using each other, but I think even NT friendships do that to some extent as NTs crave companionship just for the sake of it. (Woman with autism)

Some women have identified that there are particular types of people who appear to either be drawn to them or whom they are attracted to.

> I think there is a kind of maternal woman who tends to take me under her wing – could it be the same type of woman who likes to 'fix' men? The problem with that kind of woman is that they eventually end up bossing me around or using me for their purposes. And when I find out, it is too late; and generally what I have done several times in my life is just walk away without an explanation. (Woman with autism)

> I would attach myself to certain women in the church who seemed to be interesting or offered friendship, but it was not long before

they suddenly became unavailable or disinterested in me. (Lawson 2014, p.91)

I have one female friend as an adult who I have been friends with for over 20 years. It is likely she is also on the spectrum [...] With hindsight I think many of my male friends were probably Aspies too [...] They were all eccentric, colourful characters who were really interesting to be with. (Woman with autism)

As with their teenage selves, women with autism still find other women are not their natural peer group once they reach adulthood. I personally find their intuitive social abilities frightening – they make me feel out of my depth and more likely to reveal my social inadequacies in their presence: 'run rings round me' is a phrase that comes to mind.

I dislike other females; they are complicated and often boring. They rarely have the same interests and certainly not to the same degree. They gossip, judge people and talk crap a lot of the time. They put importance on things that don't matter, like what someone wears, looks like, social status etc. They can be competitive, jealous and bitchy. (Woman with autism)

Online friends

For younger women with autism in particular, the Internet is a great source of friendship and support, with some women saying that all of their social networks were online. This suits many people with autism as it means that they can remain in the stress-free environment of their own home, while having contact with the outside world on their own terms – it's easier to log off than to remove yourself from an awkward party scenario.

Currently, I have many friends on Facebook and for me this is an ideal medium as it saves me the awkward personal interactions. Yet sometimes I feel very lonely, with nothing but counsellors, advocates and a very distant – I mean real distance here – couple of siblings to hear me when I'm frustrated. (Woman with autism)

With regard to social media, such as Facebook, Robyn Steward (Jansen and Rombout 2014) talks about the confusion that can arise for a person with autism with the concept of 'friends' on Facebook:

> On Facebook you can unfriend a person. A lot of people on the autistic spectrum can become upset about this. They may ask themselves: someone is not my friend anymore? But a Facebook friend is not the same as a real friend. A real friend is someone who cares about you. They don't unfriend you. (Jansen and Rombout 2014, p.66)

Social isolation

Loneliness and isolation were mentioned by some women, who often found it a struggle to find like-minded companions as they got older. This was particularly the case if they had not had a long-term partner or had children. Joining groups and initiating contact with neighbours or work colleagues are simply not possible for some women – they feel intense anxiety about such things and perhaps would not even know where to begin. I know myself that I have jettisoned many evening classes and activities (French, kick-boxing) because the social requirements of the classes were too stressful and excruciating for me to contend with, despite being quite proficient at the actual skill being taught. Trying and not being able to maintain connections may feel like a bigger failure than not trying at all.

> Social isolation is not just about having mates to socialise with. It's true that if I go to the cinema, I go alone. I eat alone. I go on holiday alone and when I get home, everything is exactly how I left it. But it is more profound than that. If I am ill, no-one will bring soup or take me to the hospital. At the end of a working day, there is no-one to talk to about the stresses or the highs. If I am anxious, I stay anxious. I have no friends I can call to cheer me up. (National Autistic Society 2013a)

> At this point in my life I feel there is a total lack of friends to share interests, and that's not surprising considering my interests. I am

a 43-year-old, female, with a very niche taste (within metal music there are several dozen subgenres and I care only about two or three of these). (Woman with autism)

Animals

People aren't the only candidates to be potential friends for women with autism; animals featured strongly in the lives of some women and are generally understood to be important in the lives of many people with autism. Animals are easy to read (limited facial expressions), non-judgemental, unconditional and loyal, and have limited and easy-to-meet demands (food, stroke, walk, sleep). It is clear why people with autism often prefer animals to humans and feel that they have a real connection with them – perhaps operating cognitively in a more straightforward 'animal' way without agendas and deceit.

> I like animals more than I like people. I've always said if I meet ten dogs I'm likely to get on with 9/10; the reverse is true with people [...] I've always felt animals understand me better than people and they make fewer demands on me. I prefer my dog to my best friend. (Woman with autism)

> Animals. They are what I consider my true friends. I do indeed feel like I have a natural affinity to them, since a very tender age. I feel like I'm better able to read them than humans [...] Sometimes I do wish I were an animal, or at the very least someone who was 'as one with the wild', such as in some tribal communities, and lived a simpler yet inevitably more physically taxing life. (Woman with autism)

Enjoying aloneness

Not every woman with autism feels the need for social relationships; some are quite happy being alone, having the freedom to follow their own schedule and their own interests. Home is definitely a sanctuary for many women – a place where they can leave the persona and the internal social monitor at the door and relax. Leaving home can feel like an effort, a foray into hostile territory, and therefore some women can be in danger of getting 'stuck' in their safe place and rarely venturing out. This is fine if it is a genuine choice, but professionals need to be aware that she may need some encouragement to take a chance on the world beyond her walls.

> I like the way it's okay nowadays for people to just sit in a coffee shop by themselves. There's something nice about feeling you're part of the world and not having the stress of having to be communicating. (National Autistic Society 2013a)

> I don't really feel lost without 'friends', I don't feel like they're a requirement. It's just that it seems the right thing to do to get along life in a more neurotypical fashion; which is almost a requirement as I can't escape it. (Woman with autism)

> I'm happiest when I don't have to leave the house or see anyone. (Woman with autism)

> How peaceful it is to withdraw from the complicated world of human relationships! (Lawson 2014, p.100)

Despite continuing difficulties and social anxieties, my overall perception from my reading and experiences leads me to believe that adult women with autism often reach a place of self-acceptance as they get older. They are clearer about who they feel they want to spend time with, how often and how long for. They appear to be more comfortable with who they are, more aware of their limitations and more able to assert themselves to meet their own needs in social relationships. For some, it seems that the 'price' of certain friendships is not worth the social inclusion on offer and this realisation is a sign of empowerment and self-value. Considering the time and energy spent by these women in attempting to fit in during their teens, it is encouraging to discover that there may come a time when they stop, think and realise that their own path is the right way after all.

Chapter 10

Sexuality and Gender Identity

I very rarely feel like a woman. I feel like a man most of the time, but sometimes feel in-between, or neither, or both.

WOMAN WITH AUTISM

Throughout this book, we have mentioned the 'tomboy' profile commonly seen in women with autism and heard girls and women talk about their difficulties in fitting in with their female peers throughout childhood and adulthood. We've discussed how many are unable to identify with all things 'girly' and have a more typically masculinised, straightforward communication style. It should come as no surprise then that when issues regarding sexual and gender identity come into the picture, the logical mind of an autistic women can sometimes struggle to make sense of where she fits, who she is and who she might want to sleep with (if anyone). This sense of identity may not feel like it comes naturally and intuitively, and may have to be 'worked out'.

> [On being a woman] It's a malady I was unfortunately cursed with. I don't identify with my physical vessel in the slightest. I only see it in terms of how it pleases men; and I like being the cruel tease for fun, to snub them I suppose. It's like a tool. I think that's the simplest way to describe it. A vessel that I use to interface with the world around me, or at least try to. (Woman with autism)

It must be stressed that confusion is not the case for all women with autism; some have a clear and strong sense of their gender and sexuality, regardless of their experiences with peers. However, it does seem like a higher percentage than would be expected find themselves perplexed and alone in their feelings that they are different from anybody else out there – male or female. It is also important to distinguish gender identity from sexuality, as the two do not necessarily correlate: for example, a woman who feels more male than female is not necessarily lesbian or transgender. She may be a happily heterosexual female.

> Think more like a man, sensible, logical, even-tempered, no-nonsense, emotional level. Enjoy all things feminine, womanly (make-up, hairstyles, clothes, nailcare, grooming, decoration, cooking). (Woman with autism)

> I don't really understand the 'gender identity' concept; I have always felt female and been proud of it. I don't see gender as having an influence on my life outside of the physical/biological aspects: the differences between me and my brother relate to chromosomes, reproductive organs, inherent strength/height, and the ability to gestate a child. (Woman with autism)

Gender identity

Increasingly, as I travel across the UK and beyond, I am noticing a greater awareness among professionals of the differences in gender identity that exist within the autism population. The awareness and 'voice' of women with autism themselves also appear to be getting stronger as they find others who have spoken out and are given the courage to do the same. Many women have not been aware of anyone else feeling as they do, and therefore believe that they are odd for yet another reason. The relief of the Autism Spectrum Disorder (ASD) diagnosis can be further enhanced by learning that gender identity can form part of that profile and explain a little bit more. Women I speak to do not always define themselves in terms of neurotypical (NT), dichotomous labels of gender identity, sometimes preferring broader gender labels, such as 'genderfluid' or 'third sex'. This demonstrates the sense of not feeling either male or female, but something else.

Although individuals who define themselves in this way exist in the general population, it is among females with autism that I come across it the most. Other authors (Holliday Willey 2014; Lawson 1998; Simone 2010) have also discussed gender identity in women with autism and found a more fluid sense of belonging.

> As an adult I do not think I perceive myself as a female. Although I know I am a middle-age woman, and I am not a lesbian, deep inside I often perceive myself as a young man. (Woman with autism)

> I have often debated whether or not I am transgender in the typical Female to Male sense, but the term 'gender fluid' fits a lot more. (Woman with autism)

In Chapter 1, we discussed the work of Baron-Cohen, Ingudomnukul, Bejerot and colleagues, who all suggest that testosterone plays a part in the development and profile of autism. This leads to the conclusion (by some) that women on the autism spectrum present a less feminised profile. This has typically been interpreted as meaning that girls with autism are more masculinised. As previously discussed, Bejerot *et al.* (2012) suggest that the profile may simply be more androgynous (i.e., non-gender-specific) as opposed to specifically masculine. It is hard to perceive gender as anything but dimorphic, when perhaps what we presume to be 'more masculine' is simply 'less gendered'; hence the identification with a 'third sex' stated by some.

> When I say I don't feel like a woman, people are likely to assume that I mean I feel like a man. I don't. Never have. Nor do I feel alienated by my body, its female shape, its female cycles. (Kearns Miller 2003, p.157)

> I still see myself as relatively genderless, as I did when I was much younger. I have traits derived from both sexes but I don't fully identify with either one. It's only safe to say I lean more strongly towards masculinity than I do femininity. There has been talk of 'third genders' emerging. I feel like I'm one of them; akin to the *hijras* of India. In laymen terms I feel like a chimera. (Woman with autism)

I do not feel either. I am glad to be a woman, merely because it gives me the ability to have children which I love. I don't feel especially female, whatever that is; indeed, I have always preferred the company of men. I feel more comfortable when in a social setting with men, which is probably why I coped very well working in a prison surrounded by 1700 men. (Woman with autism)

I don't feel like a 'woman'. I just feel like a 'thing', other and alien. (Woman with autism)

This androgynous profile is described by women themselves as more masculine – perhaps for want of a better word when considering something like gender, which is typically believed to be dichotomous.

I remember saying many times during my teens that I wanted to be male in my next life. This was because their lives seemed more interesting and it seemed that they got a better deal in life. It was not really that I wanted to be male, more that I got on with them better and felt alienated from females; and also being female meant boobs and periods, smells and moods! (Woman with autism)

As far as I can recollect I have always perceived myself as a male. I cannot really describe what is it about me that makes me think I'm a guy and not a woman. It's like my inner voice is a young man. The moments when I am most at peace and enjoying myself (i.e., walking alone listening to music on my headphones) those moments I am a young man. I don't think I'm very feminine in my gestures or my intonation. I know I walk like a man too. (Woman with autism)

When I pondered on the act of sex I often felt like it was more fun from the male's perspective. Being the girl seemed boring, like a chore, rendering oneself as an object for the time being. And orgasms? I snorted at the thought of them, thinking them the stuff of myths; and I still do, having never managed one myself. I guess I'm going to come across as brutally honest here but I enjoy the thought of male on male sexual encounters in my mind. They excited me more than heterosexual interactions. In my dreams, come to think of it, I am almost always a male entity. Perhaps I really do have a secret want for being male. (Woman with autism)

As a woman with autism who does not identify with a female gender identity either mentally or physically, it makes perfect sense to me personally that individuals with autism would be more likely not to identify with their physical birth (cis) gender, or any gender, and that in some cases this is intolerable.

Transgender people

A lot of people give transwomen a hard time about their appearance or even existence. With autism, insults and criticism cut straight to the bone every time. Please keep that stuff to yourself. We're trying very hard and just want to be normal like everyone else. (Transwoman with autism)

Interestingly, despite the number of women who described their more male gender identity, the only transgender people who responded to my requests for participants were transwomen – male to female transgender people. I had no responses from cisgender females now living as men. However, I was able to speak to Wenn Lawson, a psychologist, writer, researcher, poet and academic with high-functioning autism, who has made the decision to transition from a female to a male gender identity. He told me that a psychiatrist he had spoken with had said that he had known of some individuals with autism who had transitioned and had lost their diagnosis along the way; they were able to live and function so well in their 'new' gender (with the social requirements associated with that gender) that they no longer met the autism criteria. (Lawson 2014). For Wenn, there is a distinct difference between feeling not female and feeling that you are actually male. We must remember that diversity across individuals with autism is as broad as in any other population and that not all women with autism who do not relate to typical female experience necessarily want to actually change their physical gender.

I am one of those people who, while not feeling female, have never felt that I am actually male.

De Vries *et al.* (2010) studied a group of young people referred to a gender identity clinic and found that 7.8 per cent of these individuals met the criteria for ASD. Pohl *et al.* (2014) found that women with autism show a greater tendency for 'gender dysphoria' and 'transsexualism' than NT controls. I myself have met and worked with a number of transmen and transwomen with ASD. On being asked why she thought that there were more transpeople within the autism community, one transwoman replied:

> Maybe because autistic people aren't influenced by others and are more likely to just be themselves. That's my best guess. (Transwoman with autism)

Anecdotally, it is widely believed that there are more transgender people within the autism population than elsewhere; both transmen (female to male) and transwomen (male to female). One adult Asperger Syndrome service in Brighton reports that 9 per cent of their 170 members identify as transgender, the majority being transwomen. They also report that at the time of first contact with the service almost all of the transpeople who approached them for support were undiagnosed with autism. Many stated that their gender identity issues had masked their autism. On asking those within the transgender community, I've been told anecdotally that autism is very common, although usually undiagnosed. My own experience of working with individuals with both autism and gender identity confusion leads me to believe that there is a connection between the two.

> There's certainly a connection between my autism and my transgender/homosexual stuff. They're part of my neurotype that makes me, me. I don't think they can be separated [...] As far as if I'd only had one issue or the other: If I didn't have autism, I feel I would have transitioned in my late teens. I wouldn't have let a little bad news tell me not to do it. I would have also been more self-sufficient (I never held a job for more than three months back

before my diagnosis with autism). If I'd just been autistic, I really worry I would have been one of those people commonly referred to as 'neck beards' or 'men's rights'. By being female, but having to live as male, I learned to understand both genders and their ways of thinking (typically). I really value that insight, now. (Transwoman with autism)

The strong sense of not belonging with one's same sex peers, and feeling alienated from one's birth gender is common for those with autism. Therefore it is not surprising to me that many individuals feel that their brain and body are so incongruent that they are unable to continue living within the 'wrong' body. I believe it is important to support individuals in understanding both aspects of who they are in order to achieve positive outcomes and manage expectations. Changing gender will not alter many of the challenges that an individual with autism will face and will not be the answer for some. For others, it is exactly the right choice.

One man I worked with had long-standing gender identity issues that were causing him enormous depression, anxiety and suicidal feelings. He was conflicted about whether to transition and tormented by uncertainty. He was then diagnosed with an ASD. Prior to this he had believed that gender identity had been the all-encompassing challenge affecting everything else in his life (work, relationships, mental health, sexuality), but later came to see that his autism was the main factor and that his gender identity could be explained by the cognitive and psychological impacts of his life with autism. He had previously been trying to find a place for himself on an NT gender/sexuality spectrum. I suggested to him that maybe the autistic gender/sexuality spectrum was different – more androgynous, less dichotomous, more fluid – and that his error had been to attempt to categorise himself using a system that did not apply to him. He found this reframing helpful and was able to make a decision to continue to live as man while accepting his more androgynous/feminised profile. For each person, the right path will be their own, but they may need support in finding it.

The big reason behind all this is so I can be comfortable in my skin. I've only recently started to understand how much more normal I can feel like this. I assumed all of my anxiety and awkwardness was due to my autism, but it turns out that gender was a big part of those problems, too. (Transwoman with autism)

When asked when they first had a sense of difference in terms of their gender identity, the transwomen's responses indicated that this came early in their lives – perhaps even before any awareness of their autism.

Eight is when I noticed it, but I didn't understand what it was until high school. I just didn't feel like a boy and felt disconnected from my body and felt parts of it were wrong. I have always had a very feminine personality also. (Transwoman with autism)

Around puberty, 13ish? When I saw all the girls going through a puberty that I wasn't, it just felt so wrong. I had some idea earlier, but I wasn't sure why. I always tried to play with the girls at recess, but was always shunned. I never understood why. (Transwoman with autism)

For many transpeople, the decision to come out and transition is a difficult one, perhaps made more so by their autism. Often their fears were largely unfounded and support was forthcoming.

The biggest impact was from my tendency to take everything at face value. The few documentaries I saw about transgender women always showed their lives falling apart and them facing tons of discrimination. Because of that, I hid my feelings so deep no-one had any idea. It wasn't until my early 30s that I'd finally heard so much positive about being trans that I was comfortable coming out and transitioning. Of course, my family and friends all accepted me and my wife even helped me with all the things I needed help learning. Hell, she even married me while I was fully presenting as female and we were both in dresses. I really wish I'd known then what I know now, but I trusted the handful of things I saw to be honest about it. (Transwoman with autism)

In working with young men, young women and adult women with autism, it is necessary to include gender identity in any discussion on the impact of their autism. Women find great relief in knowing that their sense of not belonging in terms of gender is also part of their autism. It means they are not alone, or at fault; it's just part of the autism deal. Supporting women with autism to accept their identity and not continuously compare themselves unfavourably with NT women or men, or dislike the less typically female or male aspects of themselves, hugely increases confidence and self-esteem. Finding resources, videos and support from other women with autism to foster a sense of belonging and community is more valuable than can possibly be imagined. An opportunity to be open about gender confusion without judgement is necessary for these individuals. Any support must also begin with autism, rather than from an NT perspective, which may be very different. Where an individual with autism feels strongly they are transgender, support should address both autism and transgender issues and needs.

Sexuality

It has been suggested that women with autism have a greater propensity to be asexual, gay or bisexual than would be expected within the NT population (Ingudomnukul *et al.* 2007). Women with autism specifically are found to 'show a significantly lower degree of heterosexuality when compared to males with ASD' (Gilmour, Melike Schalomon and Smith 2012, p.313). Others (e.g., Pohl *et al.* 2014) find similar outcomes. Within the women questioned for this book, only around 50 per cent defined themselves as heterosexual. My experience suggests that some individuals with autism can have a more blank canvas approach to sexuality and that some decide on a pragmatic basis what their sexual preference is, rather than it feeling like an innate part of who they are. My own sexuality is something I have never felt the need to define. Evidence would suggest that I am heterosexual, yet when I'm asked, I have a tendency to say that as I haven't met every person in existence,

I can't possibly know. There may be a woman/transperson/other who might sweep me off my feet, but I haven't met them yet. I have always been baffled by the certainty that most NT people appear to have around their sexuality. How can they be so sure?

> The short answer is: I'm a lesbian. But since questioning where the borderline is between male and female is my bread and butter, what it means to be attracted to women is a bit of a slippery concept. I'm open-minded about having sexual partners who are androgynous/ have different gender identities/have penises, so basically, I can be attracted to anyone with breasts and no facial hair. (Transwoman with autism)

> I always knew I had feelings for women but this never seemed a realistic thing for me, I had never met a lesbian. I was 26 when I first got with a woman and I haven't looked back since. I was never confused by my sexuality really; coming out wasn't a big deal, perhaps because I did it so late and these days most people aren't bigoted about it. Several friends had worked it out long before I did. I think I spent a long time barking up the wrong tree because that's what was expected of me and I had a series of failed relationships with men because I was aspiring to be a conventional woman, I was trying to conform to what society expected from me. (Woman with autism)

> I don't feel like a man in a sexual sense. I am not a lesbian and have gone as far as experimenting to see whether I was. I have kissed two girls, in one very drunk night, and enjoyed it as much or more than kissing a man – girls don't have scratchy beard. I have also dated a lesbian girl, got as far as having dinner and a car ride, and was revolted when she touched my leg. So that is how I know I am not a lesbian. Plus, I have this idea that a proper family requires a male and a female, so that children get the right exposure to both genders as role models. (Woman with autism)

> I wonder if my sexuality is due to my autism as I was vulnerable as a teenager and males took advantage. But I'm not sure I would be

gay if I had better skills to deal with sex and relationships. (Woman with autism)

Asexuality

One study has found that individuals with ASD show a higher rate of asexuality compared with NT controls (Gilmour *et al.* 2012); again, due to difficulties with social interaction, a preference for solo activities, sensory issues with intimacy and a different perspective on gender identity, this should come as no surprise. Around 20 per cent of the women I spoke to defined themselves as asexual. Most had felt that heterosexual relationships were something they were supposed to have and enjoy; therefore most had attempted to have these before eventually learning that it was OK not to want or like such intimate engagement.

> I think my aromantic identity has been more fluid over the years and certainly when I was in my 20s and desperate to fit in with my peers, having a romantic partner was something I believed would give me that acceptance and approval I needed. (Woman with autism)

> I just felt like a female that wasn't that interested in relationships. I never felt gay or anything. Just more interested in my hobbies and having fun in life than in romantic relationships. I always felt pressure though to be like other women and have a boyfriend and as though I was a bit of a failure because I didn't want that. (Woman with autism)

For some, the realisation that being asexual was an acceptable way to be came as a great relief, having previously assumed that there was something either psychologically or physically wrong with them for not seeking a relationship.

> At age 51, I became aware that the term 'asexual' was not just a description concerning amoebas (as I'd been taught in biology) but also a valid sexual orientation. After extensive reading of forums, blogs and a lot of honest, soul-searching about my past failed attempts at dating and relationships, I realised that the description

of asexuality as being someone who does not experience sexual attraction, fitted me perfectly. To know that there was a reason for my lack of sexual attraction to other people was a huge relief, as was discovering a whole community of people online who felt the same way as well. (Woman with autism)

I obviously wasn't normal and felt too ashamed to tell anyone for fear of them rejecting me as being too weird. I persevered with trying to mend myself by reading even more magazines and self-help books and experimenting with having sex both drunk and sober, but nothing seemed to work. I concluded that I must be the dreaded f-word, frigid, and spent years feeling broken, worthless and consumed with self-hate. (Woman with autism)

I think the keys to a happier life are awareness and acceptance (both self- and society's) of people's differences, combined with knowledge and self-understanding. If both autism and the whole spectrum of sexuality are discussed openly and sincerely in mainstream society, then maybe there will be more tolerance of people's differences and this will lead to young people having the courage to be proud of who they are and not feeling so much pressure to conform.

Chapter 11

Personal Relationships

For a very long time I believed I was a hopeless case. 'How could anyone love me?' I just wanted one person to walk beside me and accept me for who I was.

WOMAN WITH AUTISM. (HENDRICKX 2008, P.88)

For women with autism, personal relationships are as fraught with confusion and uncertainty as any other social interaction. Additionally, these usually include emotional involvement, intimate physical contact and sharing one's time, space and possessions for extended periods. Societal gender expectations lead us to believe that women are good at this stuff, that nurturing and caring come naturally and intuitively and that women who find this tough are somehow cold, damaged or just plain 'weird'. As well as all the autistic reasons that make finding, establishing and maintaining a relationship with a significant other difficult, by adulthood, women with autism have had the message hammered home that they are not ideal companions. We have heard how these women mask and hide in order to present a more acceptable public version of themselves. A close personal relationship is a place where a person ought to be able to be their true self: their best and worst self, accepted without judgement. To reveal this real self to a partner is terrifying and makes the woman vulnerable to further rejection. She may also not be a great judge of character and therefore end up making a poor choice of partner, perhaps feeling grateful that they would even bother with her defective self. The majority of women with autism seem to want a partner, with or without the sexual element, and only a few choose to remain happily single.

Potential partner as intense interest

At many points in my life I have engaged in borderline stalking of selected people who I have become infatuated with – thinking about them constantly, wanting to know everything about them, what they did and where they were, and planning how to accidentally 'bump' into them in the hope that they would be as pleased to see me as I was to see them. As a teenager, I used to cut my arms (see the self-harm section in Chapter 13) and this sometimes involved etching a boy's name into my skin with a safety pin. Once I showed one of these boys what I had done, thinking he would appreciate my handiwork and recognise my devotion to him. He was horrified and thought I was quite scary and mad. He wasn't even my boyfriend; he was just the latest target for my obsession. Thirty years later, the scars are still visible. I remember surreptitiously picking up a discarded cigarette end dropped by one object of my intense adoration, along with a coin he had given me, and storing them lovingly in a drawer in my room. I am only grateful that Facebook didn't exist in my teenage years – I would have been worse.

> After chasing him obsessively for months, he finally rebuked me in an angry, frightened voice, 'You're not a girl; I don't know what you are.' That was the first time I realised I could scare people, but I still couldn't fathom what I'd done wrong. (Simone 2010, p.80)

> If I fancied someone, I would get totally obsessed with them to the point of not enjoying life. I would sit by the phone for hours, waiting for them to ring. I would pace around the house all day with nothing in my head [but] that very person. It was well beyond the usual infatuation. (Woman with autism)

The focus of intense interest on people – rather than objects, as typified by males with Autism Spectrum Disorder (ASD) – has been discussed in previous chapters and therefore should come as no surprise.

Women with autism cannot read the signals of interest and attraction, and may struggle to perceive how the other person is feeling, which might not be as they wish.

> Of course, it's important to consider others, but all I could feel was my own need. I still find it difficult to put myself 'in the other person's shoes'. I can only feel my needs and myself – everything outside is foreign and alien to me. (Lawson 1998, p.113)

Women with autism may need support to understand these strong feelings for another person and learn how to put them in perspective and recognise them as part of their autism. A friend or mentor may need to explicitly state what socially acceptable behaviour is and what may be considered scary and weird.

> I am only just beginning to see that maybe it was my Aspieness that contributed to the failure of past relationships. I remember apologising a lot and especially saying, 'I'm sorry, I didn't think…' as I would do things which were upsetting but I didn't mean to upset them, or things would occur to me to do which I should have done. (Woman with autism)

Reading signals

The ASD profile makes reading signals tricky and this is no more evident than in the sphere of personal relationships. It's all about the subtlety, the flirtation, the unsaid. For a woman with autism this is a minefield of misunderstanding and uncertainty, which can lead to obsessive stalking-type behaviour or, alternatively, vulnerability to abuse. She cannot tell who is interested in her, or who is not. If you cannot read people's desires and intentions, things become very stressful and sometimes dangerous.

> Due to the autism I missed a lot of social signals and had no idea if or when someone was attracted to me. I didn't understand the rules of dating, despite having by now graduated to *Cosmopolitan* magazine and using it as an instruction manual for my socialising;

and to be honest, I couldn't see the point of playing games anyway. (Woman with autism)

I'm told that when younger, my inability to read signals left a small succession of men feeling rebuffed and vaguely puzzled. I'm flattered and bemused. I hope they were good-looking. Some years ago I was in a relationship. He had to practically club me over the head and drag me into the cave before I realised he was interested. (National Autistic Society 2013a)

The communication style of a woman with autism is blunt and to the point. If she wants to know if someone wants to have sex with her she may ask them outright before even knowing their name. Alternatively, she may waste no time in telling them that she will not be having sex with them. This is not how the dance of attraction is supposed to go. The intrigue, the uncertainty and the anticipation are all part of the fun for neurotypical (NT) people; not so for the woman with autism. She just wants to know. On many occasions I have been described by male partners as 'too heavy' for asking for their thoughts on how they thought the relationship would proceed – to be fair, this was sometimes on the second date. This was assumed by the men to be a sign of somewhat premature emotional attachment, which scared them. In fact, it was simply a need to know exactly what it was; I didn't mind either way, I just wanted to know. The concept of 'going with flow' and 'seeing what happens', favoured by many, was too stressful and uncertain for me.

Selecting partners

Women with autism are pragmatic creatures and may have more practical requirements from a mate, whose needs they will have to meet and presence they will have to tolerate. Sharing interests and lifestyle were important considerations for the women I questioned. Undoubtedly, concepts of 'chemistry' and 'connection' apply to women with autism when selecting partners, but this is not something that anyone mentioned.

I chose my husband because he had some amazing gym equipment I wanted to use. (Woman with autism, Hendrickx 2008, p.24)

He had an interest in virtually all of my favourite activities, even my favourite pastime that no one else had ever expressed an interest in. (Woman with autism, Hendrickx 2008, p.24)

Some women described their partners as needing to be part carer and to look after them, as they felt unable to manage alone.

Before the bizarre rush to acquire a mate, the thought of being alone didn't bother me in the slightest; if anything that made me feel empowered, like I didn't need anyone and I was a free spirit. Since after the event, and now, it's the total opposite. I question my likelihood of survival without another mate. It's not due to the craving of emotions either; no, it's just I realize more and more how inept I am at taking care of myself and at life as an entirety. (Woman with autism)

I like having a partner, as long as they are able to help me with things. Essentially, they have to be a bit of a carer for me, too, as well as a partner [...] I like having a partner but could never live with anyone. I need my own space and don't like feeling pressured or to have to be social or compromise all of the time. (Woman with autism)

I have never lived on my own for more than a few months as I really struggle, but I manage OK with a live-in partner. I have paid help with housework. (Woman with autism)

Sensory preferences may form part of the choice of a partner, which are separate from physical attraction in the typical sense. I strongly relate to Liane Holliday Willey's description of her husband Tom's face from a purely aesthetic perspective.

Sometimes all I need to keep from falling over the edge is to look at Tom's face. I am stunned by the looks of his face, not so much because he is an attractive man, but more because, in the structure of his face, [I] see so many of the visual elements that appeal to me – linear lines, symmetry, straightness, perfect alignments [...] It is a visual respite for me. I am oddly calmed when I look at his features, so calmed that I find just looking at him puts me at ease. (Holliday Willey 2014, p.95)

As expected from a lifetime of negative responses, some women did not feel worthy of having any selection criteria for a partner and were willing to go out with anyone who asked. Some described their partner choices as 'random', which is not surprising – if reading people, 'connecting' and understanding one's own emotions and those of others are all difficult or impossible to do, partner selection becomes almost a lucky-dip approach. Just like crossing roads or assessing danger, without context such decision-making is problematic.

> My boyfriends tended to choose me, rather than the other way around, and I was just grateful that someone thought [of] me [as] girlfriend material. (Woman with autism)

> I had absolutely no interest whatsoever [in having a boyfriend] during my teens. I'd grow incensed at the sight of public displays of affection, seeing it as a waste of time and a needless distraction of focus. I only started feeling a sudden desperation when I was about 22 [...] I was rather abruptly consumed by thoughts that my life would never achieve fruition if I didn't have a significant other for support. Looking back at it now, I wish I never let that feeling get the better of me [...] it's left me broken and torn. (Woman with autism)

Staying single

Some women with autism I spoke to had never had a personal or sexual relationship and others had tried (usually because they thought they were supposed to), but decided that it wasn't for them. See the section on asexuality in Chapter 10 for more on this.

> I feel sexless. I don't like sex [...] I never have wanted to have sex, ever. I did it because I thought I had to. (Woman with autism)

> I never had friends to come up to my flat or small get-togethers and now I am quite fearful of people coming to visit me. I never met a

boyfriend either but I have now accepted that I will always be single and am happy living on my own. (National Autistic Society 2013a)

For others, the lack of relationship was more troubling and they would have liked to have found a partner, but for various reasons this had not happened. It may be that they had missed signs of attraction or had not felt strong attraction to anyone themselves. What is known is that gender, sexuality and libido may be experienced differently for those with ASD and that norms in these areas should not be applied. The biggest issue for the women who had no established relationships was often a feeling of failure in an NT sense; that they had not managed to achieve what other people had in terms of finding someone who chose them as their exclusive partner. This is a very visible aspect of adult life; people around you know if you are single. Being single is often seen negatively in our society: 'no-one loves you, therefore you are unlovable'. We know that women with autism want to fit in, be accepted and be invisible. For some, not having a partner is the ultimate sign to the world that you are just no good.

> Quiet men are usually attracted to me as they see me as caring. I have never found any Asperger guy attractive, which is sad, but again I feel as though any who I would feel confident talking to would depend on me to talk for them. I've no idea why I feel this way; but I would have had plenty opportunities for boyfriends but they just didn't attract me and I didn't feel it was right to pretend that I fancied them when I didn't. (Woman with autism)

> I have never had [a boyfriend] and used to feel a freak because of this. Men would pick up that I was nervous of them and probably still do. I still feel a freak to be honest. (Woman with autism)

For transpeople with autism, living in a body that does not reflect their inner self, combined with the usual suspects of autism, may result in a reluctance to have a relationship.

> I've never been in a relationship – partly because of lack of social skills when I was at school and lack of contact with women since then

(due to hanging out in the autistic community so much), and partly because I don't want a sexual relationship until I've finished my sex change, and I've got a body that I can be proud of. (Transwoman with autism)

First sexual encounters

The range of numbers of sexual encounters reported by the women I spoke to spread from zero to more than 30. Earliest sexual experiences were at 14 years of age and many involved alcohol and some regret. A sense of gratitude that anyone would choose them, wanting to feel 'normal', plus, sadly, sometimes some naivety and coercion, can lead young women with autism into sexual encounters that are less than positive. Young women with autism are in great need of support in learning the rules of the NT world and in building self-esteem *vis à vis* a world that views them as different.

As a teenager, I thought that if someone wanted to have sex with me then it meant that they liked me. I felt intensely proud that anyone would pick me to want to have sex with. I had no idea that for many young men, there wasn't much of a selection process, and my willingness was all that was required. I also didn't say 'no' because I didn't know I was allowed to. I thought people wouldn't like me if I said 'no', and I wasn't going to risk that.

> It was quite exciting discovering sex. I remember using the phrase 'I did that!' after giving him an erection. (Woman with autism)

> I had sex for the first time when I was 16, and it was part out of curiosity and part coerced by my sexual partner. I regretted that first experience then and still regret it now. He was such an idiot, and I didn't feel anything special, other than dirty and embarrassed. (Woman with autism)

Vulnerability to sexual assault

The notion that girls and women with autism are particularly at risk from predatory individuals is well reported (Attwood 2007; Holliday Willey 2012, 2014). Misreading cues, naivety and taking what others say and do at face value can all lead to problems, particularly for a vulnerable woman. Women with autism believe what they are told and assume that other people have good intent because they themselves do. Women in my sample described themselves as 'gullible', 'vulnerable' and 'naive'. The known characteristics of autism can result in serious danger when applied to sexual situations. Many of the women I spoke to reported multiple occasions where they had been abused, attacked and/or raped. I, too, have been sexually assaulted, largely due to my autism. I was on a first date with a man I had met via Internet dating. I had gone back to his room because my favourite thing at the time was learning to play the guitar and he said that he had several and I could play them. I had carefully considered this situation and concluded that, as he had shown zero signs of interest in me (and I had none in him), this offer had no hidden agenda. It transpired that I was wrong. I can only presume I missed something somewhere, or gave him a signal that I hadn't intended. I was 35 years of age. I have an IQ of 150+. This kind of mistake has nothing to do with intelligence, but everything to do with social understanding. If you cannot determine on an individual basis who is safe and who may be a danger, due to being unable to intuitively pick up the signals and read the context of the situation, you are left with two choices: trust everyone or trust no-one. People have commented that surely I must have learned over the years, but this is not really possible. Regardless of how proficient I become at deliberately learning how people behave, I am not fluent enough to accurately predict what *that* person will do at *that* moment given *that* set of circumstances, which is why I remain terrified of people in situations where there is no context or purpose for being there (i.e. someone walking down a street behind me).

As a young woman, and because of my inability to understand social context, I was in real danger on a number of occasions; one of them in particular could have ended very badly for me. (Woman with autism)

I trusted him completely, and took his word like the gospel; he could've spirited me away to just about anywhere and my mind would be absent of any ill-intent present. I was obsessed by his countenance, at what I took to be at face value, which was probably completely the wrong impression. (Woman with autism)

I've been in a couple of abusive relationships. I'd describe most of my ex[e]s as not very nice people, but then I guess that's why they're ex[e]s. I'm not sure I'm a good judge of character. I think I've been obsessed by people and been blind to their faults. (Woman with autism)

She would say that her last relationship was at times emotionally abusive. She used to get into terrible 'trouble' if she misread something or said 'the wrong thing'. This resulted in terrible depressive meltdowns and eventually a breakdown. He ended the relationship (broke the engagement) because of the subsequent AS [Asperger Syndrome] diagnosis – [he] did not want children like that! (Parent of woman with autism)

Rape

It does not surprise me that women with ASD could be more vulnerable to rape and serious sexual attack. An inability to read and assess people and situations can clearly lead to dangerous and distressing consequences. I have often remarked that I am amazed to have made it this far without ending up in a ditch due to the many poor decisions I have made, which could have ended badly. I suspect that there are many women who have been subjected to this kind of situation, but feel too foolish and stupid to tell anyone what happened. It is hard to explain why you thought something was a perfectly good idea at the time, only realising your mistake after the event – and being aware that other people would judge you as unbelievably stupid for making the choice you did.

> My first experiences were not willing. I lost my virginity at age 14
> to my cousin [...] rape. I misread cues and ended up in situations
> where dates expected sex and I froze and could not fight them. I got
> pregnant at age 16 as a result of one of those encounters. (Woman
> with autism, Hendrickx 2008, p.82)

What I have found interesting is the way that some women with autism
have been able to get over traumatic, personally invasive events, such
as sexual attack. While rape is undoubtedly harmful both mentally and
physically, and nothing must detract from that, it does appear that some
women with autism are able to see the event quite objectively and move
on from it. It goes without saying that each individual's experience and
perception will be different and should be supported according to their
individual experience and needs. One woman with autism describes
her experience of rape and how it sits in terms of other stressors in her
life.

> Once I was raped. But this actually ranks very low in my list of
> stressful life events (so much so, that I've never bothered to mention
> it in any of my counselling sessions over the years) [...] It happened
> because of my social naiveté [...] When I realised rape was inevitable,
> I shifted goal to simply staying alive. Thus it was with a sense of
> relief rather than trauma that I survived this incident [...] On the
> other hand, a type of incident high up on my stress list involves the
> difficulties of communicating with co-workers. I am still as helpless
> as ever at dealing with this sort of thing. (Kearns Miller 2003, p.243)

Liane Holliday Willey (2012) recalls a number of incidents of sexual
assault that occurred due to her naivety. She talks about needing
to carry out 'cognitive restructuring' to understand and look at the
events in a more positive way. I use a similar approach using basic
cognitive behavioural techniques (CBT), which can be found online
and in CBT books. I am loathe to recommend anything specific as
different people favour different approaches, although for me as a
practitioner and for personal understanding, I have yet to find anything
as well written as *Cognitive Behavioural Therapy for Adult Asperger*

Syndrome (Gaus 2007), along with its companion workbook *Living Well on the Spectrum* (Gaus 2011).

Other women describe ways in which they have learned to protect themselves following difficult experiences with potential partners.

> [I] listed 10 qualities I wanted in a man. Sounds strict, but had to set limits for myself to keep from being vulnerable. (Woman with autism)

> Life has not led me to think that my own feelings and emotions are valid or meaningful, so I use others as a yardstick for knowing what is acceptable. (Woman with autism)

Sex and intimacy

In my previous book on sex and relationships in ASD (Hendrickx 2008) I noted that women with autism were more likely to see the emotional and physical side of sexual interaction as more separate from each other than was generally expected in NT women. Often their perspective was closer to what is often perceived as a more male approach to sex. Many of the women questioned for this book expressed similar thoughts. For some, the presence of a partner for meeting sexual needs wasn't required at all.

> Libido was like an itch that needed scratching and the most effective method would be to satisfy it myself by masturbation. The connection here with my autistic traits I feel is that interacting with another human requires more effort (also more stress and anxiety) and the outcome is not as predictable as going solo, as it were. Obviously, there is also my requirement for space and solitude, and if sexual satisfaction is all that is required at that time, then why complicate matters by involving someone else? (Woman with autism)

Women reported confusion about the concept of intimacy and emotional connection. Some said that they didn't feel it at all, and others felt it very strongly but not necessarily in relation to physical sex. For me, sex feels like a tangible, concrete way to connect with my partner.

I don't know that I understand the concept of emotional closeness – it's too vague, too abstract – but physical closeness is a means of feeling safe with someone when at your most vulnerable and most 'naked' self, which I think, for me, is as good as it can get.

> I am still very confused about the connection between intimacy and love. I tend to view sex as a basic animal instinct, a need that has to be satisfied, like hunger or sleep. When I have sex with my husband, I do not like to think of him as my husband, the person I share my life with, and who I have a child with. (Woman with autism)

> What the body needs and what the spirit needs is different at different times. (Woman with autism, Hendrickx 2008. p.90)

> I am not capable of telling if the other person has an emotional attachment to me or not, but as long as I do then sex can proceed. (Woman with autism, Hendrickx 2008, p.91)

The sense of 'connection' for some women did not come from sexual interaction, but from companionship and intellectual sharing – something more mentally nourishing, rather than physically so.

> Having sex with a person I love does not make me want to connect on an emotional level with him while I am having sex. It is as if sex is too functional, too dirty, and why not a bit risible and over-dramatic, to smear it on someone I care for. I prefer the foreplay, kissing, hugging and caressing. And as for connection, I'd rather connect with my loved one through the mind, through sharing ideas and activities, and through comforting physical contact. (Woman with autism)

> I have to have some manner of bonding with the person before the thought even emerges about allowing that person access to my nether regions. The thing is though, sex is not a priority; I could quite happily get through life with someone I genuinely liked without having sex. What I desire the most is mental mutuality. Once that is there everything else falls into place. (Woman with autism)

Successful relationships

Women with autism tend to form relationships either with others with ASD (Hendrickx 2008; Simone 2010) or with those far on the other end of the empathising spectrum (teachers, nurses, counsellors, carers). In male/female relationships, the most common pattern is a double ASD partnership. In same-gender relationships, either extreme can apply.

> I once thought I was incapable of falling in love with someone and connecting the way that others seemed to. My partners were chosen at random. Just in the past two years I have learned that I am capable of forming a connection. Curiously enough this connection is with another individual who has AS. I wonder if that is part of what made it possible. (Woman with autism, Hendrickx 2008, p.47)

The partner is often the best friend and only person required in the woman's life. Her social and emotional needs may be fairly small (in comparison to an NT woman) and are most easily met by a partner with similar requirements. Men with ASD may be attracted to her for the same reasons she is attracted to him: shared interests, intellectual knowledge and an appreciation for a direct and straightforward approach (no game-playing, no mind-reading). For women with ASD, NT men and women may be too socially complicated and emotionally demanding, expecting intuitive empathic reading of emotions and requirements that are beyond them.

> Relationships are still so demanding, so confusing. I want to relate to other people but I'm not sure I can survive the pain of it all. Some days my brain is so sore from trying to work out what it is I am supposed to do or to say, that I just cannot do it for very long. (Lawson 1998, p.97)

> My relationship is crucial to me; my partner is also my best friend and constant companion. I am loyal and faithful; I don't see any other male as attractive or of sexual interest when I am in a relationship. My partner feels like part of who I am. I don't miss him when we are apart – I can often forget about him completely when I'm busy

at work. Neither of us knows when the other is wanting sex and neither knows how to initiate it, so we have somehow developed a routine to approaching it, which sounds boring but it isn't; it totally works for us. (Woman with autism)

I have a belief in an intuitive ability that I call 'Adar' (in reference to the reputed gay radar, 'Gaydar', where gay people can spot another gay person purely by sight), by which individuals with ASD are drawn magnetically to each other without any conscious thought. My partner, Keith, and I met online. Neither of us knew that the other one had ASD when we started to communicate, nor for several years afterwards. We are two peas in a pod, delighted to have found each other after many failed attempts. How on earth we managed to find each other, I don't know. I put it down to Adar. We do not require anyone else in our world. We can happily spend 24 hours a day together for extended periods and not get irritated or overwhelmed (as is the case with every other human being in the world). We place few emotional demands on each other and any that are placed are explicitly defined, avoiding uncertainty, anxiety or potential for failure. Most importantly, we accept each other without judgement, regardless of how odd and unfathomable our behaviour is. As a woman with autism, this has been a once-in-a-lifetime experience for me, a respite from the performance I put on for the rest of the world, a place to truly call 'home'. I cannot emphasise strongly enough what a difference this has made to my entire life.

I think my husband and I get along very well. I don't think I have ever had such an honest relationship as I have with him. With other partners I always felt as if I was acting. With him is like taking my shoes off. When she first visited us, my mum was surprised as to how well we got along as a couple, considering we seem to interact so little. (Woman with autism)

My husband is my rock; I really don't think I could go back to being on my own. I have become reliant on him to support me. I cannot believe that I coped for so long independently before I met him. I do believe that if he hadn't come into my life I would have committed suicide. The level of exhaustion I felt was awful. I sometimes wish that I had never met him, because not only have I trapped him, but I have trapped myself by having children who really need me. (Woman with autism)

A good partnership can provide a woman with ASD with the acceptance and support to reach her potential in other areas of her life. I know for myself that before meeting Keith I spent all of my energy and capacity in trying to fix bad relationships – changing myself to fit what other people told me I ought to be – which left me mentally and physically harmed and incapable of pursuing things that might make me feel good about myself. It is no coincidence that everything positive I have achieved has happened since I met him. Women with autism need support in recognising a nurturing relationship and identifying what that looks like for them. It is important not to judge how people live and to support women to work out what they require to make a relationship manageable for them. Unconventional set-ups might be the answer for some: co-habiting might not work (Keith and I lived more than 50 miles apart for the first nine years of our relationship); sex might not be a requirement and separate rooms may be a necessity. Unconventional people require unconventional solutions to conventional arrangements. What is clear is that many women with autism are living happily in relationships with their partners and families.

Chapter 12

Pregnancy and Parenting

Having a child is said to be an enriching experience for any parent. For me this enrichment came two-fold: as a woman, and as an autistic woman.

MOTHER WITH AUTISM

Parenting as a woman with autism has, until recently, been a concept largely overlooked. Despite knowing that autism is an inherited condition, the assumption has perhaps been that – in line with the 'males get autism' default – children were getting it from their fathers only. All of the features of autism that affect individuals – good or bad – on an everyday basis, also affect them as parents. For some women, it is a relief to know that they can do something right after all.

As an autistic woman, becoming a mum taught me an immense lesson in empathy, tolerance and care; a lesson in love. I learned that I can successfully ensure the survival and well-being of a creature who depends 100 per cent on me. Now I know what it is like to love someone, I can apply that to other people, and I can measure, I can classify, I can understand the process of love and what is involved. Being a mum has made my emotional life much, much richer, and much clearer. And knowing that I am an Aspie mum, who can empathise with her autistic child like no other mum could, makes me feel empowered, and confident that I can raise a happy human. And that is no mean feat. (Mother with autism)

> It's a great ongoing project that allows me to research things, obsess, and shop online. I would say my baby is my new special interest. (New mother with autism)

Children are, after all, people. Having autism generally means that relationships with people are frequently disappointing, confusing and draining. It would be no surprise then to discover that women with autism would not want to be virtually attached to another person all day, every day for a number of years of her life, but that is not *always* the case. Regardless of the feelings involved in the decision to become a parent, women with autism need support for the duration of the journey. Parenting is not easy when you are neither socially intuitive nor flexible.

> Babies have round-the-clock needs. They're stressful, messy, unpredictable and demanding. Basically, they are everything that an autistic person finds hard to cope with. Gone was my precious alone time. Gone were my carefully crafted routines. Even my body was no longer my own, transformed first by pregnancy then by postpartum hormones and breastfeeding. (Kim, in Hurley 2014, p.26)

Wanting children

I have met many women with autism who have absolutely no desire to become a parent, as well as individuals who have been obsessed by the idea from an early age. Some of us take on this role more by accident than design. I never wanted nor planned to have children, but I ended up with two; my mother felt the same and had three. The concept of women with autism as mothers (often of children who also have autism) is largely overlooked by research, support and society in general. This is, I suppose, initially due to the 'only men get autism' viewpoint along with a perhaps mostly unspoken and maybe unconscious perspective that people with autism don't do relationships and wouldn't have children or be very good at taking caring of them. Around half of the women questioned for this book had children. Most had at least one child with an Autism Spectrum Disorder (ASD) and/or other developmental conditions. Research has suggested that women with autism have a lower interest in marriage and children than neurotypical (NT) women (Ingudomnukul *et al.* 2007) and this was certainly mentioned by some of the women in my sample.

> I never craved marriage or children and saw much female behaviour as silly and disempowering. (Woman with autism)

> [No interest] whatsoever: maintained my entire life that I was not having children – even when we got married. (Mother with autism)

Others had a very strong yearning to have children for one reason or another.

> I always had a desire to have children. I wanted to be married and have five children. As I got older and not yet married, my number wished for got a little smaller […] one of each sounded pretty good. (Mother with autism)

> Someone else to focus on. I hope it will make me less self-obsessed. (New mother with autism)

> I've always wanted to have a child, but was always too afraid of childbirth itself growing up; and then after I was diagnosed I was afraid that I wouldn't manage with the constant presence of another person, given how draining I find people. (Mother with autism)

Pregnancy

> [Pregnancy was] very planned, with military precision. I bought lots of things like [a] thermometer and ovulation test strips, and made a diary, and read up on the fastest way to get pregnant. It only took three months of trying. (Mother with autism)

Pregnancy is an exciting and overwhelming experience for any woman, but for a woman with autism, the experience may be somewhat more intense. She will have to cope with feeling completely out of control of her body, which changes almost by the day. She also has little control over the process that needs to be adhered to. There are appointments, new people and plenty of physical contact from strangers: both those needing to perform examinations and random strangers who feel that touching a pregnant women's stomach is acceptable behaviour. She may not have a social peer group of friends who are pregnant at the same time, or have been previously. This can make this an isolating and frightening time, with no-one to share worries with.

> Pregnancy was terrorising the first time. I was all of a sudden AFFLICTED by pregnancy and therefore not the owner of my body any longer; nothing was within my control, and it was awful, just awful, not knowing how it would end. (Mother with autism)

> I have said in the past – to the horror of my listener – that pregnancy was the worst time of my life. It was really hard to see my body change shape so quickly. My usually dodgy balance and lack of spatial awareness made it very hard for me to move without knocking something over or falling or banging my limbs somewhere. The worst of it was, perhaps due to lack of social imagination, I didn't know whether at the end of the ordeal I was truly going to love my baby as everyone else seemed to think – I was too terrified of being judged so I kept my fear to myself. (Mother with autism)

> If I had had a full diagnosis – not just a suspicion – that I had AS [Asperger Syndrome] when I got pregnant, perhaps the whole experience of spending ten long months of uncertainty, which led me to depression, would have been different. (Mother with autism)

Typically, some women with autism take on pregnancy as a special interest and devour every scrap of information that they can on the subject.

> It was very exciting to find out I was pregnant. I was looking forward to it all and scared at the same time. I wanted to know how to do everything. I read every (literally EVERY) publication that I could find on what to do during pregnancy and how to take care of a baby and child. It was very helpful to take away my anxiety of doing

everything right. I think, for the most part, I did know what I was doing. There was some confidence that came with all that reading. (Mother with autism)

Personally, I loved being pregnant because I liked being special, and it was easy to chat to people because they only wanted to talk about one subject – me and my expanding belly. I had horrendous morning sickness during both pregnancies but otherwise I was fit and healthy, stubbornly refusing to moderate my exertions and behaviour throughout. My son had to be induced after a particularly vigorous evening of dancing at a wedding made my waters break. I took my driving test at 36 weeks pregnant with my daughter and was still working as a lorry driver with my father at the time. I never felt in any way maternal or feminine.

For those supporting women with autism through pregnancy, it is important to provide clear information about the processes that they will be expected to go through and also opportunities to ask questions. They may not have any peers who have been through the experience to talk to. When making a birth plan, consideration should be taken with regard to sensory issues, such as physical touch, pain thresholds and communication approaches.

> Asperger women report the need to feel more empowered about their birthing day and their experience is reliant on three factors including: clear communication, sensory adjustments and change management. (Autism Women Matter 2013)

Giving birth

All of the information-gathering, mental and physical preparation and planning during pregnancy are the build-up to the actual giving birth. For the woman who prefers a schedule, the realisation that giving birth quite frequently does not go to plan (despite her meticulous efforts) and that the process is likely to be out of her control – either by nature or medical intervention – is an utterly terrifying experience with no known end point.

What is the purpose of a due date? I think you should have a due month, much less specific! When my due date came I sat at home waiting. Nothing happened and I became highly agitated and upset. I paced around the house wondering why nothing was happening [...] I couldn't process the fact that what was supposed to happen obviously wasn't going to. (Grant, in Hurley 2014, p.66)

After the delivery, I withdrew. I curled up into a ball and tried to comfort myself by sucking the roof of my mouth. The nursing staff left me alone and I slept on until the early hours of the next morning. When I awoke, I remembered I had a baby and I knew I needed to act like a mother or else I might lose him. (Lawson 1998, p.80)

Autism Women Matter (AWM) (2013) conducted a survey with mothers on the autism spectrum and found that their birth experiences had been affected by the lack of support for their autistic needs. The whole experience of giving birth is extremely overwhelming for a woman with autism, who may feel completely terrified about the huge range of stimuli – both internal and external – that she is required to tolerate. It also may be the case that she does not behave in a way typically expected of a woman about to give birth. She may be particularly quiet because she doesn't know what she is expected to do or ask for, or alternatively she may be extremely distressed if touched, for example. Comments about their experiences of giving birth from those surveyed by AWM include the following:

Communication issues

During birth, [midwives and doctors] need to be more reassuring and explain each stage clearly to reduce anxiety. (Autism Women Matter 2014)

Please explain clearly that a new midwife is taking over your case and not just leave and a new one walks in. (Autism Women Matter 2014)

I was told to push again for next delivery; when I asked why, they said 'second baby' and laughed – they meant placenta, but I was terrified as I thought they meant twins. (Autism Women Matter 2014)

The main thing was that they didn't believe me when I said it was nearly time to give birth. I didn't make any noise and was so quiet going through contractions that they said I couldn't be anywhere near ready. When they checked, I was fully dilated and had to be taken straight down to the labour suite. (Autism Women Matter 2014)

Sensory needs

People coming in and out of the room were disruptive. I ended up locking myself in the bathroom in the dark for eight hours of my labour. I had the same repetitive soothing music on for pretty much the whole labour. (Autism Women Matter 2014)

The ward was hell on earth. I can't sleep with strangers in the room so I was awake all night, and my baby screamed all night. None of the midwives helped me. I hated the noise, the chaos, plus my vomit phobia meant my anxiety levels were through the roof. (Autism Women Matter 2014)

They dimmed the lights for me and let me play the music I wanted, even though it was 80s pop instead of calm music. (Autism Women Matter 2014)

I had a home birth with two private midwives; I was well supported. I felt safer and more comfortable at home, rather than going to hospital with strangers and bright lights. I did a lot of research [...] I had my son by candlelight, my husband in the pool with me. Sensory wise I didn't want to be touched unless I asked for it; I also didn't want talking, and I had quiet music. (Autism Women Matter 2014)

Breastfeeding

Experiences and feelings about breastfeeding varied in the women I spoke to. My own experience of breastfeeding both of my children was unsuccessful. I didn't know how to do it. My mother – who possibly had ASD – had not been successful at breastfeeding her three children and so could not advise me; furthermore, she was not particularly encouraging because she could not see why it mattered anyway. I had no peers to ask and thus gave up after a few weeks in a state of exhaustion, misery and failure. I did not know where or how to get help. I did not know what was normal, what I should expect and whether I was doing it wrong. All I knew was that no matter how long my babies fed for (hours and hours at a time), they were still hungry and still crying. It felt like breastfeeding was something that ought to happen naturally but it didn't. I had no emotional, nurturing urge to breastfeed; my only rationale for doing it was that I had read that it was the 'right thing to do', which led me to persist. The experience was painful and distressing for both me and my babies. I had to be persuaded to give up by my partner, who was concerned for my well-being, because I couldn't bear to admit defeat. Other women found it a more nourishing and supported experience, which should be the case for all women who wish to breastfeed.

> I loved having that time to just sit and be with my baby. It gave me the excuse to have time out from everyone and everything and just sit and be still with my child. (Autism Women Matter 2014)

> I was lucky to be in a room on my own with just a nurse to check on me and help the babies to latch on. This really helped me from a sensory point of view. (Autism Women Matter 2014)

> My mum didn't breastfeed because she found it too painful. I am feeding my baby with expressed breast milk using a pump because we were unable to establish breastfeeding directly. My baby wouldn't latch on, and it was important to me that she had breast milk. (Woman with autism)

I fed both of my children. I made it my life's duty. I fed my eldest for 3½ years and my youngest for 4½ years. That's eight years between them. (Woman with autism)

If a woman wishes to breastfeed, she should be supported to do so, but may need additional help in working out how she will manage sensory issues and in understanding her baby's needs if these are not obvious to her. She may need to ask many questions and be shown several times what to do. It should not be assumed that this understanding is implicitly or intuitively known as this may not be the case. It is important that she does not feel judged or a failure as a mother for not finding it easy. Guidelines suggested for supporting breastfeeding among women on the autism spectrum include:

- Use of visual instructions and diagrams.

- Direct verbal communication approach.

- Avoid innuendos and metaphors.

- Be aware that individual support may be preferable to breast-feeding groups.

- Verbalise your intent to touch if needing to make physical contact.

- Consider reluctance to try a new approach as potentially temporary; the mother may need time and supplementary information in order to embrace changes. (Pelz-Sherman 2014)

For those who choose not to breastfeed, equally they should not feel judged or guilty for not 'doing the best' for their baby. If it is simply too uncomfortable or stressful for a woman to feed her child, she may be doing more harm than good by persisting. The well-being of the mother generally best supports the well-being of the child.

Being a mum with autism

'Why can't you be like other moms?' That hurt. I'd be singing opera very loudly in the car. Apparently other moms didn't do that. (Simone 2010, p.140)

The experience of parenting is life-changing and all-encompassing for any woman. For a woman with autism, additional challenges arise. There are expectations for socialising her child, birthday parties, school meetings and playing, all of which mean not having much time to herself, which may be crucial to her functioning and well-being.

> Truthfully? Loathsome, and with little return. Both my children have autism as well, and it's been grim – fighting for diagnoses, fighting for education, fighting with the LAs [local authorities] for provision, etc. It's like a constant fight that you can't back out of, and it never ends – it's always time for the next Annual Review or IEP [Individualised Education Programme] meeting or Phase Transfer. (Mother with autism)

No-one knows how many mothers with autism there are and what impact this has on them and their children, as it has never been studied. The Autism Research Centre in Cambridge has initiated a study of mothers with autism at the time of writing (December 2014), so recognition has begun. The impact of mothering and how mothers with autism are perceived is one that UK-based advocacy group Autism Women Matter is bringing to public attention.

> My baby doesn't have a routine yet, so it makes it hard to plan a day. I've found people want to make plans with me, but that it's even harder than it used to be before I had a baby, and I struggled then with social commitments. I'm encouraged to go out and go to groups, neither of which I enjoy; but I feel I have to so that my baby doesn't miss out. I seriously struggle with the lack of sleep as I don't function without sleep and it makes my depression worse. The hormonal changes have hit me hard, too, and I am now well medicated. I resent the fact that I am clumsier and more forgetful than I was before I was pregnant, and I get frustrated with myself when I knock things over or lose things. (New mother with autism)

> It's so hard! My partner keeps saying he told me it would be hard, but there was no way to prepare me, no way to explain what it's like. I regretted it in the first few weeks after she was born because I

thought I couldn't do it, but it's getting easier. I seem to be linked in with lots of support services now because I've been very open about how hard I'm finding it. (New mother with autism)

Many women writing on the subject of parenting with autism describe feelings of inadequacy, and thinking that everyone else is doing a better job than they are.

I still feel the pangs of sheer inadequacy. My peculiarity will smash me in the face time and time again and I think 'What the hell am I doing raising kids? I'm no mother at all'! (Kearns Miller 2003, p.195)

Other mothers had more money, more patience, more stability and never seemed as stressed as me. They talked to each other in the playground, they met each other for coffee. I was never invited. (Simone 2010, p.140)

I often marvelled at these women that I knew who would go out in the evenings to shop or socialize or attend events with their children. I crashed. (Kearns Miller 2003 p.215)

I became pregnant at the age of 18 after a drunken one-night stand. I was a gifted child from a perfectly ordinary working-class family, who, despite the high hopes and support of everyone around me, struggled to reach my potential at a very good school (part-scholarship), had no interest in university or a career and started to drink a considerable amount of alcohol at the age of 14 to achieve a 'normal' social life. By the time I became pregnant with my first child I was working part time in a pub and drinking half a bottle of gin a day, having previously lived in squats since leaving school at the age of 16. I often say that having a child saved my life and I believe that to be true: it gave my life both function and structure. I now had something to do. I took motherhood very seriously and wanted to do it to perfection. Parenting to me has been a project like any other with outcomes to be successfully met. My views of bad parenting remain vehemently strong; I think it is one's duty and obligation not to harm a person that one chooses to bring into the world. I feel that I have failed substantially to be a perfect parent, although this is partly because in the early days I didn't know that this isn't possible (or so I'm told). I tried very hard to get it right and continue to do so. I'm not the only one:

> Despite trying very hard, I always had the sense that what I was doing was never enough. (Simone 2010, p.140)

One of the biggest challenges I have faced with my own children has been in judging abstract situations such as discipline and danger. It seems to me that other parents have a degree of certainty that their opinions are correct on many matters, whereas I could only assess a situation on the basis of logic, rather than 'because I said so' or any other hierarchical or social basis. If my children asked if they could do something, mostly I couldn't see any reason to say no. I didn't mind them going out with no shoes on in the rain, wearing odd clothes, or eating dessert without dinner – I couldn't really see the problem. In order to determine what was generally acceptable and safe behaviour, I closely observed other parents to see what their reactions and decision-making processes were, frequently asking questions such as, 'So what time does John's Mum think he should be home?' and based mine on theirs. I gathered a database of parenting skills from other people because I was unable to accurately assess individual situations by myself – they were too abstract, with too many variables. I lived in constant fear of my stab-in-the-dark risk-assessment process. (I use the same approach when crossing roads; I am unable to process all of the data available and so just step out hoping for the best. I receive more toots of the horn than most.)

I discussed things with my children as equals and perhaps expected too much emotional maturity from them in return as I was disappointed when they were unable to behave in what I considered to be a reasonable manner. I was devastated when they lied because I couldn't understand why they would do such a thing. It felt like a baffling personal attack from someone who was supposed to love you; my chest physically hurt when this happened. My parenting style was extremely lax in many ways because many things seemed irrelevant and unnecessarily restrictive to me. I couldn't justify making a rule which had no firm, evidential basis for it, even if it was my preference. I worked from logic rather than ego. I home-schooled my daughter and took her to work with me on a campsite in France because she was unhappy in what I considered to be a negative and self-esteem destroying regime in her village school. I shaved my son's hair into a Mohican for him as a teenager (because I knew I could do a good job, having had one myself). In other ways, I am fiercely rigid and strict; respect, manners, not causing harm or inconvenience to others, and taking responsibility for your actions are all of supreme importance to me. I rarely shout as a parent, but rather tend to become silent (and apparently terrifying) when angry or upset. This is mistaken as a brooding type of anger, but it's simply because I don't have the ability to process my feelings and articulate them; I just feel a whirl of emotions and physical sensations: dizziness, nausea, tight chest and overwhelming emotional pain – no words would come close to explaining how I feel. My children say that what they hate most is when I show my disappointment in them. I don't mean to be disappointed (and fail to conceal it), but my standards are unreasonably high – for myself and the rest of the world. Rudy Simone (2010) describes mothers with autism as 'unconventional yet conservative moms; strict, safe, logical, protective and intellectually stimulating' (Simone 2010, p.140).

Sometimes I think that my enjoyment of my children has been overshadowed by the sheer effort of parenting. For me, it has been a feat of endurance and obligation. It is only since they have grown up that I have enough space to actually see them properly (they're quite nice and very beautiful). I see other people having the capacity to enjoy being a parent in a relaxed and easy way that I have never experienced. They actually seem to like it. I am known to stare at these women with incredulity and some sadness.

The greatest emotion I feel in relation to my children is protection: if they are wronged in any way, I rear up like a lioness, snarling and fearsome in their defence, in complete contrast to my usual 'wouldn't say boo to a goose' personality. My strong sense of justice and defence of the little guy shows itself most strongly when it comes to my kids. When we go paintballing and one of them makes a run for it, I am on their tail blasting the enemy into paint-splattered oblivion. (We women with autism never grow up, either.)

> I hope that, when I don't show my love for them in the more traditional ways that other parents do (it has been pointed out to me, for instance, that I seem to hug and interact with them less), they still recognize my love for them in qualities like the determination with which I stand behind them through thick and thin, like the fierce mother defending her young. (Kearns Miller 2003, p.199)

On many an occasion over the years, I have stopped and explicitly contemplated the thought that I have two children; and every time I struggled to fully comprehend how that could possibly be the truth. It has never ever sunk in. Despite having been utterly overwhelmed by the experience of parenting for 27 years, I hate to think what would have become of me had I not had something so important to do, which gave me routine and structure in my life. There is a good chance that I would not be here for one reason or another, given the path I was on. I actually have no idea what people without children do with themselves. I'm not sure how I'd have coped with such a fluid existence.

Other mothers mention the intrusion and difficulty involved in tolerating their child's friends visiting the house, as having any person in their homes is something that many find a challenge, let alone a noisy, messy, irrational experience. I always dreaded having other people's children in my care, out of fear of something bad happening to them that would be my fault, and for not knowing how to talk to them. The weight of the responsibility was too much. I always found other people's children far more irritating than my own, who were intelligent and sensible. I have always been extremely gullible and believe whatever I am told, so cannot judge when anyone has a hidden agenda. My six-year-old grandson has better theory of mind than I do and can use this to manipulate me. I am fortunate that my children did not take more advantage of this.

The mothers with autism in my survey are often aware that their children have more to tolerate than their peers. 'Coa' writing in *Women from Another Planet?* compiles a list, from which the following are an abridged selection:

- A mother with extra-embarrassing habits, such as lack of make-up, hairy legs and who is liable to appear in public still in bedroom slippers with pen in mouth.

- A mother who cannot model social skills (beyond her level, which they have surpassed).

- A mother with annoying and unpredictable processing delays and requirements [...]

- A mother who provides a largely asocial environment, with rarely anyone here besides us, because that's how I need it to cope [...]

- A mother who requires them to take on adult roles beyond their years [...] (Kearns Miller 2003, p.203)

I have been terrified of my children (and others in my care) coming to harm, every moment of every day, and it being due to some oversight of mine that anyone else would have seen coming. Liane Holliday Willey expresses a similar thought:

> The parents I know seem to have the same kinds of experiences to recount and the same kinds of problems to relate. My worries and blunders come from places they do not seem to know exist [...] This used to bother me tremendously. It used to make me feel I was incapable of being an acceptable mom. (Holliday Willey 2014, p.99)

I have also been terrified that at any given moment, I might get it wrong and I might be found out to be the inadequate mother I know I am. My own diagnosis of autism came when my children were almost adults themselves, but I certainly wouldn't have told anyone for fear of being considered an unsuitable parent. It seems that I am not alone with these thoughts.

> The con that worries me is that perhaps somehow I could be seen as a worse mother if I officially have Asperger's, I know it doesn't make me any worse of a mother but I worry that somehow it could be used

against me and I don't trust Social Services to understand Aspieness. (Mother with autism)

As my children grew older it became more difficult to cover up my sense of inadequacy. (Lawson 1998, p.87)

I love them dearly and they have kept me going when I wouldn't have bothered, but being what is expected as a 'good parent' has broken me in ways they will never know. (Mother with autism)

Some women feel that their autistic personality has provided them with positive abilities as a parent. It is likely that there may be a lot of reading involved with an autistic mum (Simone 2010) – which should come as no surprise – as well as colouring, learning and 'doing' activities. I could never engage in pretend play with my children, but would happily build Lego® and train sets alongside them. However, it is fair to say that I tended to take control of the activity and tried to insist that it was done my way. I loved colouring, cooking, and teaching them about nature and other countries, but was never able to show my daughter how to put on her make-up or advise her what to wear! I have never missed my children. I said this to Wenn Lawson who admitted to feeling the same and what a relief it felt to be able to say it out loud (Lawson 2014). It's the thing you are not supposed to say as a mother; that you can love them, but function quite happily without them and not need them to make you feel whole or indispensable.

Other women felt that their autism brought a positive sense of rightness to their abilities as a parent, which came over as a sense of pride and determination.

As a woman with autism, I can focus on what is really important. I always put my kids as a priority in my life. I wanted them to have what they needed in material things and in their environment, like I did growing up. (Mother with autism)

My determination to do it RIGHT, as is defined by myself. (Mother with autism)

There is some advantage in having a mother who does not project her own needs and wants on her children, and who just accepts them for who they are. (Kearns Miller 2003, p.212)

I spent lots of time with the children. It was a very safe place to be. It did not matter whether I played games with them on the floor, did finger-painting, played with home-made playdough or joined in hide-and-seek, they never said I was dumb or stupid. (Lawson 1998, p.85)

I'm very organised, because I have to be. I already use lots of lists and reminders, I'm good at sticking to a schedule; we always have food and nappies in the house. (Mother with autism)

Being mum to a child with autism

Those women with autism who had a child with autism spoke of a special bond with that child and of having the intuition to know what their child needed even when it was different to what all the books and advice stated.

I never felt alienated from him. I never felt this abyss that many NT parents of autistic kids say they feel between them and their autistic child. (Kearns Miller 2003, p.212)

I love being able to really understand my kids. (Mother with autism)

In Adrian's case, the books were wrong. Any baby care book that doesn't include the topic of over-stimulation is not credible. (Kearns Miller 2003, p.195)

I have a personal crusade to get kids who have certain social issues tested and, if relevant, diagnosed with autism. I don't understand the denial of certain parents; it makes me very angry. Perhaps this is even caused by my own faulty social imagination. Because as soon as I saw what I thought were signs of autism in my son, I had him diagnosed. I faced the facts, and I live with them, I don't understand denial. (Mother with autism)

Children of autistic mothers

I did not interview any children of mothers with autism regarding their experiences as a child of an autistic mother, although a number of the women I spoke to believed that their mothers probably did have ASD. Due to the ages of the adult women (and therefore the ages of their mothers), it was usually the case that they had not broached the subject with their mothers. It would be interesting to ask children with autistic mothers for their experiences.

> Good decisions based on sound theory and information doesn't exactly have a motherly ring to it but the practice mothered Adrian well. In living an AS life, I have collected abundant personal examples of using alternative means to good result. It's still very difficult, though, for me to override the cultural belief in a socially sentimental and intuitive form of loving as the single, legitimate source of parenting. My mother-love is deep and passionate, but it's really quite useless! (Kearns Miller 2003, p.195)

Overall, we could summarise that women with autism make perfectly good mothers, but often do things in their own unique style. It is perfectly possible for them to produce children who feel accepted, listened to and valued for who they are; children who are allowed to be independent and find their own way; children who accept difference. My kids are certainly quirky in their own way; they are opinionated, confident and generally good people, but both are totally messy despite my best efforts. It would be interesting to study the children of autistic women and see if they follow any patterns – perhaps this style of parenting has advantages. For the majority of women, parenting doesn't appear to come naturally, but their way with logic, trial and error and commitment appears to compensate quite nicely.

> I certainly don't mother the way most women mother. My affect may still be flat as a pancake on too many occasions (though I've taught myself to smile more and laugh more and touch more), but I know something now. I think I do. Maybe I do. It appears likely that I'm a good mother, a loving mother. How very peculiar! (Kearns Miller 2003, p.195)

Chapter 13

Health and Well-being

I feel unwell most of the time; either a headache, stomach ache, feelings of anxiety or general fatigue. They're nothing serious, but there's always something that means I feel less than 100%. Simply existing just seems to be hard work.

WOMAN WITH AUTISM

Physical health

Due to the almost complete lack of research to date focusing on women with autism, the nature of any associated physical or mental health issues specific to this group is unknown. In my experience, and from the responses provided, it would appear that women with autism experience many different health difficulties. I have been called a hypochondriac due to my never-ending list of 'niggles', as I call them: aches, pains, intolerances and sensitivities that affect my everyday life, and I can see that the same could be said, incorrectly, of other women with autism. Some of these diagnoses preceded the diagnosis of autism and may now be understood as facets of the autism profile, rather than distinct conditions. Some are self-diagnosed and others may be incorrect diagnoses; for example, Obsessive-Compulsive Disorder (OCD) is sometimes wrongly diagnosed in an individual with autism when the observed behaviour is simply a need for structure and routine, rather than an irrational or compulsive thought. Obviously, how each person experiences and perceives the symptoms of these conditions varies between individuals.

Dyslexia, dyspraxia, Mears–Irlen Syndrome, generalised anxiety disorder, clinical depression, Obsessive Compulsive Disorder, endometriosis (severe), asthma, partially sighted, Irritable Bowel Syndrome, Raynaud's syndrome, allergies. I think that's everything! (Woman with autism)

Learning disabilities, dyslexia, ADD [Attention Deficit Disorder], Scotopic Sensitivity Syndrome (visual perceptual problems), asthma, Irritable Bowel Syndrome (gastrointestinal issues), hypothyroidism, neuropathy, migraine disorder, depression, and anxiety disorder. (Woman with autism)

Asthma, chronic non-allergic rhinitis, IBS [Irritable Bowel Syndrome], ME [Myalgic Encephalomyelitis], migraine, synaesthesia, RSI [Repetitive Strain Injury], chronic daytime sleepiness, depression (recurrent depressive disorder, I think), anxiety, PMS [Premenstrual Syndrome], hypoglycaemia. (Woman with autism)

Hypermobility issues in back and neck (confirmed by chiropractic practitioner), dyscalculia (undiagnosed), depression, trichotillomania (very mild now but quite pronounced in teens, flares up with stress) and generalised anxiety. Eating disorder issues (under-eating and over-exercising, but not anorexia). (Woman with autism)

The impact of these conditions is all undoubtedly real and I have never yet met a woman with autism whom I believe to be fabricating their health concerns or making an unnecessary fuss. If anything, the opposite is true: these women are often just getting on with life in considerable discomfort and pain, without seeking medical help. The hyper-awareness and detail-focused nature of a person with autism perhaps means that these women may notice more acutely when something doesn't feel right. Women with autism can turn themselves into the focus of an intense interest and become their own project. They are often experts in their own conditions and should be involved in decisions relating to any treatment process. If they do seek medical advice, it is likely that they will have researched all possible options and may even know more than the practitioner about specific conditions. Rather than become defensive about this amateur clinician, health care professionals would be wise to listen and take note; the woman may well be right and save the practitioner a lot of time.

It is clear when looking at the responses quoted here that the conditions that featured most regularly have a singular root cause: stress. Many of the physical conditions experienced by these women are manifestations of a body and a brain that are overwhelmed: migraines, Irritable Bowel Syndrome, specific and generalised anxiety disorders, Chronic Fatigue Syndrome (CFS, also known as ME) and fibromyalgia are all reported by individuals and support services as anecdotally mentioned by women with autism. Liane Holliday Willey (2012) goes so far as to state that her gastrointestinal doctor believes that stress led to the loss of her gallbladder and removal of most of her sigmoid colon. These are the consequences of living in a world that is unknown, unpredictable and unsafe, both socially and physically. In treating and working with women with autism, we must take the autism into account when proposing treatment; it may be that the best 'cure' for some of these physical ailments is in supporting a greater self-understanding for the individual, which will allow her to know her limitations and assert herself in making them known to others. I know for myself that it has been literally life-saving for me to understand how limited my capacity is compared with others, and that regardless of how it appears, it is essential for me to limit my activities and put my own health above appearing 'normal'. I also have to ask those around me to do the same on my behalf when I am unable to do so due to my own urge to do everything. This process is also a painful one, as it means accepting limitations and 'inadequacy' (in my mind).

Allergies, intolerances and sensitivities

It is widely recognised, and now included in the DSM-5 diagnostic criteria for Autism Spectrum Disorders (ASDs), that individuals with autism experience differences in tolerance for various stimuli. Traditionally, we recognise these to be related to external sensory stimuli such as light, sound or smell, but experience tells me that women with autism are affected by a much wider range of substances than that. Chemicals, medication, caffeine, fabric and other widely used substances cause physical reactions for many women. Air fresheners, fluorescent lighting, air conditioning, perfume, wool, aspartame, sucralose, sugar and washing powder are just a few triggers that are all around us and make life just that little bit more difficult for me personally (resulting in frequent migraines); as with physical health conditions, our reactions can make us appear to be fussy hypochondriacs, when, in fact, the sensitivity is very real.

> I have sensitivities and allergies to various antibiotics which also make my neurological and digestive symptoms worse, even after I am no longer taking them. (Woman with autism)

> I am [...] very sensitive to various fabrics which can cause redness, tiny red dots and itching. All my clothes have to be washed in liquid, fragrance-free laundry detergent. (Woman with autism)

> In addition, I am [...] very sensitive to airborne chemicals such as smoke, toxic gas, scented candles, chemical scents, etc [...] Cigarette smoke in particular causes burning in my nasal passages, throat and eyes and often causes migraines. (Woman with autism)

> I am easily overwhelmed with crowds and noisy or busy environments. I am often made fun of at work because of my compulsive tendencies regarding protecting myself from germs and from items that I feel are dirty or that have germs. I use hand sanitizer a lot. I also have problems with lighting conditions such as bright lights or fluorescent lighting, which make my visual aberrations much worse. (Woman with autism)

Mears–Irlen Syndrome/Scotopic Sensitivity

One condition that was frequently reported is Mears–Irlens Syndrome (otherwise known as Scotopic Sensitivity), which affects visual perception and light and contrast sensitivity. I could not find any research to suggest that autism and this condition are specifically linked, but a quick Internet search brings up many hits which almost take for granted that they are. Specialist opticians are able to diagnose Mears–Irlen Syndrome and provide individually tailored coloured lenses in glasses that can relieve many of the symptoms. Migraines, headaches, eye strain, fatigue, light sensitivity and visual disturbances when reading text on a page that shows high contrast (e.g. black on white) can all be consequences of undiagnosed Mears–Irlen Sydrome. It may be necessary to view symptoms in clusters, rather than as individual complaints.

Menstruation

In the group of participants that I questioned for this book, there were no significant differences either in the age of starting menstruation or in menstrual irregularities or difficulties, than would be expected from the general population. However, some research has different findings: Ingudomnukul *et al.* (2007) found that significantly more women with autism experienced irregular menstrual cycles, dysmenorrhoea and Polycystic Ovary Syndrome (PCOS), and made connections with elevated testosterone levels in individuals with autism. They found that almost twice as many women with autism experienced PMS than non-autistic controls. Another study (Pohl *et al.* 2014) found that women with autism showed higher frequencies of epilepsy, PCOS, atypical menstruation and severe acne than the control group. PCOS was mentioned by a number of the women I questioned as being something that they had been diagnosed with and this does appear to be a relatively common feature for women with autism. The exact frequency cannot be estimated as it is likely that there are a significant number of women who have undiagnosed PCOS.

Eating disorders

> Possible anorexia in my late teens and early 20s. Certainly very
> preoccupied with counting calories and exercising. It was something
> I could achieve at a time when I didn't seem to be able to achieve
> much. (Woman with autism)

Some research suggests that the cognitive profiles of individuals
with anorexia and those with ASD are markedly similar except for
differences in empathy scoring (Oldershaw *et al.* 2011). It has been
suggested that anorexia is 'the female Asperger's' and that up to 20 per
cent of individuals with anorexia may also have an ASD (Joss 2013).
'Females with anorexia have elevated autistic traits. Clinicians should
consider if a focus on autistic traits might be helpful in the assessment
and treatment of anorexia' (Baron-Cohen *et al.* 2013).

Similarities in emotional regulation and recognition, rigidity and
obsessional thinking are seen between the two groups. It may also be
the case that girls and women with autism are strongly affected by the
media's portrayal of apparently successful females and seek to emulate
this in their body size in order to achieve social acceptance. The streak
of perfectionism that most people with autism admit to may also play
a part in these women aspiring to an unrealistic and unhealthy goal.
For some women, seeking sameness and solutions that do not require
ongoing processing and decision-making may also be appealing and a
means of managing the multiple demands of life.

> Living on bread and apples was an affordable diet and it was one
> less complication to have to deal with. The option of not having
> to maintain variety is very appealing and I still struggle with that
> today [...] I still think the monotony feels safer than having variety
> because there's less information to take in and it's easy to predict.
> (Woszczylo, in Hurley 2014, p.51)

Depression

Depression was mentioned by around 50 per cent of the women questioned, and from my experience I would suggest that this figure is likely to be even higher across this population. The experience of feeling different, excluded and living in an unjust world, yet having no means to fix things, is so common to people with autism that many perhaps do not even relate to the term 'depression' – it's just 'life'. Many women with autism I have worked with describe themselves as having been 'depressed forever' and that their low mood is simply a consequence of their limited social acceptance and daily challenges; they were unable to differentiate their depression from their autism. Problems with identifying emotional responses (alexithymia) from physical sensations can form part of this difficulty as they may not actually know how they are feeling and/or be able to articulate that into words. I also wonder (partly from my own perspective) whether having lived with a constant sense of low mood and stress for most of one's life results in someone not actually knowing what 'OK' feels like.

> Depression since mid-teens. I feel it has limited my efforts to improve my situation […] It's difficult to separate the impact of depression from that of Asperger's – I think the two have combined to isolate me for decades. (Woman with autism)

> I believe my depression is often triggered by an increase in anxiety and may be an effort to slow down and tone down the feelings of anxiety to the point that I think I no longer care about my well-being. I also frequently perseverate or fixate on issues that are bothering me in an effort to try to understand and resolve disturbances. However, often, this tendency and inability to stop thinking about issues has probably worsened my depression. (Woman with autism)

> I guess I have never lost hope that things will improve, however difficult, which I know is different to the classical description of depression. I feel like my depression is different to how other (NT) [neurotypical] people describe it. (Woman with autism)

Some women found that medication helped to lift their mood, but others had learned strategies to cope with this intrinsic part of their lives. They were stoic and aware in their responses about how to get themselves through it. Confidence in professional help was low, with most feeling that they were not understood by mental health professionals, whose knowledge of autism was perceived to be basic or non-existent. The women who had sought professional help tended to be those who had reached a very serious level of depression and saw it as a last resort.

> Learning to recognise when I am depressed is important, as it is insidious and can creep up unnoticed over a period of weeks or months. Once I notice I am depressed, sometimes it helps just to throw in the towel and 'nurse' myself for a couple of days by resting/eating as much as I feel like and having a break from normal activities, before coming up with a plan of action and getting back to a pattern of healthy activity and diet (although gently!). (Woman with autism)

> I need not to be nagged, not to have too much noise, not to be told that I have nothing to be depressed about and I should pull myself together. I actually tend to avoid people because often their reactions are unhelpful. I know how to get myself through it and would rather do it alone. (Woman with autism)

Anxiety

Anxiety is widely recognised as being a normal part of life for many people on the autism spectrum. We have seen previously that women with autism are in particular danger of being diagnosed with a mental health condition *instead* of an ASD (rather than *as well as*), and so we may conclude are more likely to present the symptoms of anxiety than males with autism. Anxiety was mentioned specifically by around 50 per cent of the women I questioned and is featured in most books written by and about women with autism (Holliday Willey 2001; Lawson 1998; Nichols *et al.* 2009).

The anxiety is an everyday chronic problem that is greatly worsened under stressful conditions, often at work or in tense social situations. Since I tend to deteriorate under pressure (or have a meltdown more or less), I now also fear or have anxiety about not being able to handle future situations. (Woman with autism)

It makes it difficult to plan things because sometimes I feel like doing something when I arrange it, but then on the day I can't face it. I let people down a lot and cancel things a lot. (Woman with autism)

Anxiety can be crippling and all-consuming if someone makes things harder for me by failing to do something or lying. I don't feel depression as such but I can get very down, again, when people make it tough for me. (Woman with autism)

Women with autism feel anxious because they live in a world that is endlessly confusing, illogical and frustrating, and full of inconsistencies and alterations to the status quo. This is perhaps exacerbated by the gender expectations placed on them, which they feel unable to meet. The result of all of this is sometimes avoidance of certain situations as well as a general sense of worry that can be triggered at any moment. The following are some of the circumstances that the women with autism found particularly stressful.

I have to avoid situations that often contribute to my anxiety. I particularly get anxious when I am alone in crowds or in crowded situations or when I have to negotiate difficult social situations. I generally need some guidance, coaching or feedback to help me deal with and interpret these situations as a lot of my anxiety results from my inability to process information in real time. (Woman with autism)

Relationships and not getting them or getting it wrong [and] the worry that goes with it. Failure is a killer. (Woman with autism)

Socialising, meeting new people, going out at night, going to parties, talking to strangers without alcohol, going to London for a night out, going to new places, birthday parties. (Woman with autism)

Meeting someone I know but not that well suddenly on a bus, [at] a bus stop, in a cafe etc. I find it very stressful trying to think what to say. I'd rather speak to someone I don't know at all. (Woman with autism)

Self-harm

People self-harm in different ways and for different reasons. We have mentioned in the sensory section of Chapter 8 about finger- and skin-picking, scratching, rubbing and plucking hairs. How an individual chooses to frame these behaviours is a personal one, but perhaps the line between a sensory comfort and self-harm is a blurred one. Mothers of girls with autism report self-harm as being of particular concern (Stewart 2012). My understanding is that girls and women with autism self-harm as a means of feeling something real (pain) in times of overwhelming emotion. Liane Holliday Willey (2012) describes her own 'scraping' as a means to reconnect with herself, but cautions that others will assume that you are trying to hurt yourself rather than trying to (in some way) heal yourself.

As a teenager, I cut myself, a lot. My weapon of choice was a safety pin. I would rub the open end over the skin on my hands and arms repeatedly until it bled and then continue to do so. I also etched boys' names and initials into my hands. I can still see faint scars now. I spoke about this at a conference for women with autism and afterwards a woman came up to me and asked to see my scars. I showed her and then she showed me hers – almost invisible names on her hands in the same place (at the base of the thumb) that mine were. We laughed. Even from our darkest moments, there is connection and understanding without judgement from others who have walked the same path.

At the time I had no idea why I did it. I knew nothing about autism. I knew that I felt overwhelming physical sensations that welled up inside my body like a volcano with no vent, no outlet for release. I couldn't attach any words to my feelings and, put simply, I didn't know what to do with them. I couldn't speak about them as I had no words for them. This is called 'alexithymia'. Breaking my skin and channelling the feelings into physical pain somehow diverted my attention into something solid and tangible and made them dissipate. There was a sense of relief and calm. Even now in my 40s, the urge to cut myself is strong at times when I feel overwhelmed. My ability to articulate or tolerate extreme emotions is no more advanced than it was at 15, but my ability to understand the consequences to myself and others of cutting myself has increased. My partner and family would be alarmed and completely fail to understand and those who employ me would be concerned about the suitability of such a person. It would be visible evidence of my inability to pass as 'normal' and, as such, harder for people to ignore, although it is simply a different way of processing sensations than is perceived as typical. For others, alcohol and drugs may fulfil a similar function by blocking out emotional confusion and the feeling of being overwhelmed. Research into substance misuse in those on the autism spectrum is virtually non-existent. I co-wrote a book on the subject (Tinsley and Hendrickx 2008), which presented evidence to suggest that social anxiety and alcoholism may be connected. Sixty-five per cent of individuals entering alcohol treatment centres have a diagnosis of Social Anxiety Disorder.

Meditation, self-awareness and, certainly, diagnosis of ASD can all help girls and women to understand why they feel the way they do and raise awareness of how to manage it safely without causing physical harm. Telling a woman to stop self-harming without supporting her reasons for doing so is unlikely to be successful and more likely to make her feel like a failure for being 'found out' as not coping.

Suicidal ideation

It has been suggested that individuals with ASD may have suicidal thoughts and make plans for ending their own lives with greater frequency than would be expected in the general population (Cassidy et al. 2014). This study found that 66 per cent of adults with autism had had thoughts about ending their lives. I was interested to know whether this was something that women with autism could relate to, as this was very much my own experience and one I have spoken about publicly.

> My Aspie opinion of suicidal thinking is [...] maybe just a non-emotional, logical analysis of the situation: suicide is genuinely one of the potential options. I think neurotypical people can find suicidal thinking very shocking [...] whereas for some of us it's almost part of everyday life. (Hendrickx, in Wylie 2014, p.111)

Other women shared their recollections and thoughts about this topic. What comes across is pragmatism about the issue and the proposed solution. I wonder whether there is a difference in the emotions and thought processes involved in suicidal ideation for those with autism in comparison to neurotypical (NT) people. This is a yet unstudied area.

> I remember deciding that I would kill myself if I wasn't happier by the time I was 25, but had no specific measures for that happiness nor any specific plan in mind. I have occasionally considered suicide over the years, but I wouldn't say I have ever actually been suicidal. When I have thought about it, it has taken the form more of how I would organise things so as to minimise the trauma for others – write a letter to the police notifying them so that my body can be found by them rather than an acquaintance. (Woman with autism)

One woman articulated very clearly her conclusions about her own suicidal ideation and how this could apply to others with autism. She also beautifully advises how this could be avoided for future generations.

> I do believe that we (autistic individuals such as myself) are very susceptible to suicidal thinking for multiple reasons that include: chronic high levels of anxiety, tendency to fixate on or get stuck on negative disturbing thoughts, low self-worth, inability to have significant or intimate relationships with others, replaying over and over again negative statements that others have said to us, feeling unable to be understood, lack [of] a solid self-identity, difficulty with expressing self to others, feelings of great isolation, feeling that you are or may be a burden to others, feeling unable to contribute

to society or the greater good, etc [...] I do believe that the most important thing that someone else can do for a struggling autistic individual is to affirm their self-worth, recognise and validate their struggles and affirm the things that they do that are greatly valued by others. The worst thing to do for an autistic individual, or any struggling individual for that matter, is to not believe them or to deny the validity of their struggles. My greatest and deepest hurt is that doctors, family members and important others did not believe me in my struggles, particularly when I was younger, before my diagnosis at the age of 35 years. This has been the strongest impetus for my feelings of unworthiness and suicidal thoughts. (Woman with autism)

In the black-and-white cognitive processing world of autism, where multiple alternative strategies can be difficult to generate, suicide may be one of the few options that the person has found. It is certainly an option that comes to my mind very quickly when considering solutions to overwhelming situations, but it is simply that: one of a number of options logically analysed and (until now) discarded as not the optimum choice at the time. Cognitive behavioural approaches that assist in perspective shifting and broadening may be helpful in supporting women with autism to come up with a greater number of options and assess their suitability. An autism-specific approach is required, that is, one that recognises both the experience and the cognitive processing style of a person with autism, rather than generic, emotion-based therapeutic intervention.

I've been in and out of cognitive behaviour therapy for 40 years and while it has helped me deal with many issues, I have yet to find the key that will lock stress out of my life. (Holliday Willey 2012, p.63)

Treatments and strategies

Medication for anxiety, depression and migraines had been helpful for some of the women with autism in the survey. I have not discussed individual medications as I feel this would be inappropriate: clinicians must make their own assessments based on the individual. I am also not knowledgeable enough to comment. Therapy received mixed reviews, with some finding it very helpful and others less so. Those who described positive support appeared to have received input that was directive and supported the learning of social understanding, rather than a more psychoanalytical, emotional 'talking' approach. An understanding of autism is crucial when considering any therapeutic support.

> In my late teen years and early 20s, basic talk therapy did not seem to be as helpful since I did not seem to have the insight (regarding my feelings and the feelings of others) necessary to benefit from therapy, and my therapist did not recognise my autism condition (I was not diagnosed at that time). He seemed puzzled by me and did not seem to know how to help me. (Woman with autism)

> My current therapist has been the most helpful to me since she understands my autism condition fairly well and she understands the need to help me with interpreting various social situations. She also has gotten me involved in music activities with others, including jamming with other musicians on a weekly basis and participating in a monthly drum circle. She has also gotten me involved in meditation activities and occasional rhythmic dance activities [...] These activities have also helped me to recognise and see that I am a worthy person with many strengths and perhaps even gifts (so to speak). (Woman with autism)

> I need their support and acceptance of what I am feeling, a willingness to try to understand me and my situation, and some coaching or guidance to help me process or properly interpret the difficult situation while helping me to come up with some resolution strategies. (Woman with autism)

> Counselling – had quite a lot, which helped at the time, but then the benefits stop as soon as the sessions stop. Some counsellors have been useless with me, asking me about my feelings, but my current one has a thorough understanding of AS [Asperger Sydrome] and

doesn't ask me about my feelings unless I bring them up, which is much better [...] I need other people to be understanding and not get annoyed with me. I need my partner to put up with being shouted at when he doesn't really deserve it. (Woman with autism)

For the most part (perhaps due to a lack of confidence in clinicians), women with autism find ways to manage their own well-being as best they can in the circumstances. Their awareness of their autism and its negative impact on their health and well-being is key to them being able to develop practical strategies for themselves.

Often, I find that the only way to relieve disturbing thoughts or fixations is to engage in positive fixations such as [...] my music, photography and art videos. (Woman with autism)

Exercise has been a great daily activity to ward off stress and tension. (Woman with autism)

Time and someone being kind and understanding when I can't cope or become overwhelmed. (Woman with autism)

Company, but understanding company. (Woman with autism)

My own therapy of writing stuff down, like encouraging thoughts, plans, notes on how to deal with people who upset me, etc. (Woman with autism)

I try to keep fit and have taken up roller skating. Walking helps with my depression a great deal. (Woman with autism)

I am very driven to create or indulge in creative activities where I can express myself, and I have found such activities and therapy to be vital for my mental health. Without such, I tend to engage in very negative self-condemning thoughts and sometimes suicidal ideation when depressed. I now recognise the triggers and I try as much as possible to avoid them and do my best to engage in positive activities and to maintain my commitments to others. I work very hard at trying to improve myself and maintain my well-being. (Woman with autism)

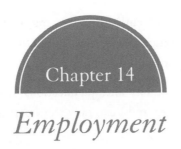

Chapter 14

Employment

I think that I've managed to struggle by in employment for so long because I became so good at faking it. In fact, over the past few years this has caused me a lot of anguish because it had got to the stage where even I no longer knew who was behind the mask and I began to fear I was going mad because I just didn't seem to know who I was anymore.

WOMAN WITH AUTISM

It is widely believed that individuals with ASD have difficulties in both obtaining and retaining employment for a number of reasons, most of which relate to their autism. There are several books on this topic, including one I have written (Hendrickx 2009), but these are all gender neutral. Work is probably the single greatest challenge for women with autism due to the long-term nature of the social relationships that are developed – you have to see the same people every day – and the sheer effort of having to be somewhere, often surrounded by people. I have had over 30 jobs, which all ended for one reason or another: my inability to cope with injustice, feeling unliked, my inability to tolerate certain people in authority whom I did not respect, not seeing the point, being inflexible to ways of doing things other than my own, and sometimes just trying to do a job that was completely outside my (what I now know to be) autistic profile. My financial situation has been extremely precarious for most of my adult life, due to my poor work record. Success in employment involves immersion into a neurotypical (NT) world for most of your waking hours. This can be a social step too far for some women with autism and they may end up working in jobs below their ability and/or unable to work full time, therefore reducing their income. Being smart is not enough.

> I work below my ability and qualifications to reduce the amount of stress I am under, and I can only work part time. (Woman with autism)

> I find the office politics a bit of a minefield, as well as the social graces and 'brown nosing' to get on rather than being judged on capabilities. I have tended to do menial jobs and was self-employed for 16 years. (Woman with autism)

> My lack of ability to bullshit or big myself up, and my poor interview skills hold me back. I am very able but do find that I think differently to others, which can lead to misunderstandings. (Woman with autism)

Challenges at work

One of the difficulties mentioned by the women I questioned related to information processing and multi-tasking. It is presumed that women can manage multiple instructions and conversations, and take on board new information quickly and flexibly. This is not always the case for women with autism, who may be very adept at structured, linear tasks and information, but take longer and require more detail for abstract information (such as directions and procedures).

> I often felt as though almost every member of staff [was] giving me instructions and often one would be telling me to do the opposite of the other. I often felt as though I was on the receiving end of many people who saw me as their opportunity to be in control […] I was slower than other members of staff at understanding things and therefore more at the mercy of every person in a workplace who dreamed of being a boss. (Woman with autism)

> I am new to office life and I feel with most things it starts off well but then you are expected to master everything. I am still getting lost in

the building and asking questions about things others are clear on. (Woman with autism)

Women with autism often have a strong sense of fairness, justice and a desire to abide by the stipulated rules. This can bring them into conflict with colleagues who may not be doing the same. This can cause enormous stress, which may make the woman leave the employment, or result in her displaying her blunt, outspoken side. A woman with autism may not be able to 'keep quiet' if she feels that a situation is plain wrong. Office politics and 'sucking up' to the boss are not in her social tool box and this can cause others to dislike her socially, despite her being skilled at her job.

> My tolerance for insincere people is very low as well as my ability to take everyone's case on board and fight their battles. Unfairness is probably my main hurdle. My complete honesty and bluntness don't seem to be an attribute in climbing the career ladder. (Woman with autism)

Gender expectations

There are specific situations in some workplaces where women are generally expected to take on certain roles without question. Women with autism may not naturally step into this role or even know that it is expected of her. We are often gender-blind in this respect and expect everyone to be treated equally, not seeing invisible gender expectations of tea-making for visitors, gift-buying for colleagues' new babies and general gossip. Even if these roles are explained, it is likely that a woman with autism would question their validity, or reject them in a direct manner, potentially causing herself to be seen as 'difficult'.

> Of course, being a woman, I was born knowing how to make the perfect cup of tea or coffee [...] However, what they don't bank on is my rubbish short-term memory [...] by the time I've reached the kitchen I've forgotten the ratio of coffee : tea : milk : sugar. (Woman with autism)

Adjustments

Disclosing a disability, should result in adjustments being made to accommodate that condition. Disability and equality laws differ from country to country, but this is beyond the scope of this book. Information on the rights of disabled employees should be sought from relevant sources in order to ensure that legal obligations are met by employers. Many women choose not to disclose their Autism Spectrum Disorder (ASD) to employers for fear of discrimination, as not all employers are open to supporting staff to perform to their optimum capability.

> I have not been able to acquire the accommodations that I need in the work environment. In fact, asking for accommodations has usually angered my employers, who don't understand me, don't understand autism and actually seem to resent my asking. (Woman with autism)

> On a few occasions people in charge of me would write instructions down or try to make them easier to understand and I appreciated this a great deal. (Woman with autism)

When disclosure is received positively and adjustments are made – often quite small ones – women with autism can achieve success at work and maintain their well-being.

> I do receive support and adjustments – I don't have to go to conferences or do public speaking, and people weren't allowed to move my desk without a lot of warning and consultation when reorganising the office. I am very open about having an ASC [Autism Spectrum Condition] at work and that takes the pressure off me as I don't have to pretend so much to be something I'm not. (Woman with autism)

> I have now found a role where I've developed confidence in my abilities because I receive positive feedback. People appreciate my attention to detail, and I enjoy repetitive routine tasks that other people don't seem to like doing, e.g., filing, categorising, routine

correspondence, setting up systems, proofreading. I work hard and I work all the hours I am paid to. I only chat to colleagues if they initiate it, and I don't go for cigarette breaks or stand around the water cooler gossiping, or whatever you're supposed to do when you work in an office! (Woman with autism)

Ideal job

Considering the difficulties of employment for women with autism, I was interested in knowing how these women felt they would perform best. Self-employment, part-time, home-working and working alone featured most frequently in the responses of the women questioned. There was no mention of earning large incomes or achieving a high-status career position by anyone. It appears that spending your days doing something that does not exceed your limitations is the priority for these women.

Many facets of their ideal job choices mirror my own working life, which I have whittled into something that I can just about manage, but eventually will need to reduce even further due to the continuing physical and mental health effects of stress. I am self-employed, spend most of my days alone, have no ongoing daily social relationships to maintain and get to take as much time off as I wish (with the accompanying lack of income). The life I am working towards involves goats, sunshine and probably considerable poverty, but at least my head will be calm. Other women expressed their own requirements.

Flexible part-time hours. Two reasons for this: one is because physically I get exhausted having to interact with people for long periods of time and need a quiet place and solitude to recharge my batteries. Second, I need to have time to pursue my own interests outside work because, again, this is how I re-energise myself and reduce my anxiety levels. (Woman with autism)

One woman had some much more specific job roles in mind:

Ideal job would be something involving the Discworld® – either creatively or at the Discworld Emporium shop in Wincanton. Failing that, then working in or owning an independent bookshop (specialising in sci-fi/fantasy – maybe like the Forbidden Planet bookshops in London), animal sanctuary (Monkey World in Dorset, or one involving donkeys, dogs or otters or other marine life), or some sort of environmental conservation (woodlands or coastal) or a nursery (for plants, not children!). (Woman with autism)

My own autism and employment research (Hendrickx 2009) found that individuals with autism are most successful in jobs that play to the strengths of their autism and minimise exposure to the differences, rather than trying to squeeze a square peg into a round hole. This seems to be confirmed by the women who responded to my questionnaire.

Chapter 15

Ageing with Autism

We simply do not know what autism spectrum conditions look like in older age [...] We don't know whether particular sorts of physical health problems are greatly raised. We should suspect that they would be because living with stress, living with anxiety, has a proven link with, for example, heart conditions.

FRANCESCA HAPPÉ (NATIONAL AUTISTIC SOCIETY 2013B)

At the time of writing, as far as I am aware, there is no research on ageing and women with autism. In fact, there is little research on ageing and anyone with autism. Research funding desperately needs to be made available to assess the impact of autism on this group.

The first generation of children diagnosed with autism in childhood during the 1940s are only now approaching their elderly years, and in light of this the National Autistic Society has developed the Autism in Maturity project to address the issues that these individuals may face. It is not only those diagnosed in childhood who make up this ageing autistic population: 71 per cent of individuals with autism over the age of 55 received their diagnosis in the past decade (National Autistic Society 2013b).

I have read books by other Aspies and trawled the Internet forums. There is a lot of emphasis on young people with autism. I was never a young person with autism, as I had no idea I had it. I was a young person with problems. I am now a middle-aged woman learning for the first time to recognise my problems as Aspie problems and look for interventions. I have the problems, but there don't seem to be any interventions available to people of my age. (National Autistic Society 2013a)

Given that around one-third of the participants in the research for this book were in their 40s and above – and most of those were only diagnosed in the last few years – we have a population of women moving towards their elderly years, the majority of whom have only just discovered who they are.

I did not know that I had autism as a child, young person, teenager, young adult or middle-aged person. That has been all a process of retrospect, of looking backwards in dozen upon dozen 'aha' moments. Some are kind of numbing to think about. Life might have been easier with some kind of intervention on my Aspie behalf. (Woman with autism, aged 62 years, diagnosed aged 56 years)

I would have liked to have been able to speak to more women in their 60s and above, but sadly few came forward to volunteer, despite my best efforts. It is probably the case that women in this group are even less likely to be aware that they have autism than younger women. Perhaps they are also less likely to take on board this information even if it were presented to them, coming from a generation where such things didn't really exist (especially for intellectually able people and for women).

We know that in general terms we are an ageing population and that support and services for growing numbers of older people will be increasingly necessary in years to come. What we don't really know is what impact ageing has on people with autism. I was interested to hear what reflections the women had on living with autism along with the natural physical and mental effects of ageing. I wanted to know whether they felt that the impact of their autism changed as they aged: Did life feel easier or harder? Did they feel 'more' or 'less' autistic in their behaviour?

Life with autism is more difficult as I get older. I realise that life as anyone gets older is more difficult. Instead of just letting it happen and be poorly adjusted to, why not strive to make it the best transition it can be? A positive outlook and some good choices can make the difference. Decide to be a role model to younger people and people with autism. They need to know that getting older can be a good thing. (Woman with autism)

These insights are important because, in stating the obvious, every autistic girl will eventually become an autistic older woman, and if we know what to watch out for, we can start the process early to minimise the negative effects.

Diagnosis of older people

Diagnosis may be more difficult for older people because they may not have living parents or family members to provide additional information relating to the childhood impact of autistic characteristics, which are required by some clinicians. I have worked with individuals who have been refused diagnosis on the grounds that they do not have a surviving parent. *The NICE Guidelines* (National Collaborating Centre for Mental Health 2012) state that, 'where possible', a partner, family member or carer should be involved, but the lack of this information source is not grounds for refusing a diagnosis.

For those who do have living relatives, these relatives are likely to be very elderly themselves and may be unable to contribute. Other people may not wish to discuss the diagnosis with elderly parents for fear of upsetting them. Individuals may also have difficulty remembering significant details of childhood events and motivations and therefore struggle to demonstrate their early development. Current diagnostic tools are largely designed for the diagnosis of children and are therefore not appropriate for older people. Care must be taken when making a diagnosis of older women to take into account that they may have successfully developed compensating and masking strategies to hide their autism. Extensive experience of working with adults with autism is required to confidently and accurately diagnose older people and be able to 'see' the autism beneath the constructed social facade.

Some people question the point of diagnosis in later life, feeling that if a person has managed this far, then they can't be very affected or need a diagnosis.

> Getting a diagnosis is very difficult as there seems to be a school of thought that if you've survived with AS [Asperger Syndrome] into your 40s, it can't be that bad (in fact there can be an enormous amount of suffering in silence). (Woman with autism)

We have heard from many women of the benefit and relief that a diagnosis can bring. These women feel a sense of who they are, of belonging somewhere after feeling that they didn't really belong anywhere; not with men or with women.

> For over 50 years I thought I was defective. This tells me I wasn't defective. It makes all the difference to me and means I can start asserting myself and asking for my needs to be met. I've never been able to do that before as I thought it was me that was defective. (Woman with autism)

> It's getting easier, mainly due to having been diagnosed and [seeking] information about the condition. For most of my life I had no clue I had AS and was really handicapped by it in many ways. Life experience has helped a great deal – I think those of us with AS can learn and improve our lives, but it takes longer than it does for most people and we need to have things explained to us that most people seem to pick up instinctively. (Woman with autism)

Accessing health and social care

Individuals with autism are known to have differences in the way that they experience and report pain (National Autistic Society 2013b). This may mean that they do not alert professionals when they are unwell. They also may have more limited family and social networks, which may mean that their poor health goes unnoticed for considerable periods of time. For non-verbal individuals with autism, this difficultly can exhibit as challenging behaviour and the underlying health problems go unaddressed. Care must be taken to ensure that older people with autism are sufficiently monitored, particularly if they live alone in the community.

> I don't experience pain in the same way as other people [...] I can open up the oven, pick up a cast-iron casserole, stand up with it, put it on the table, and it's only when my niece says, 'Auntie, your hands are peeling off,' that I think, 'This isn't good', but it'll be another five minutes before mild discomfort becomes agony. I missed appendicitis completely and woke up in hospital with peritonitis. (Nancy, National Autistic Society 2013a)

Accessing health care for individuals who experience anxiety and difficulties with new situations may be exacerbated in older life when accompanied by dementia, hearing loss, memory loss and poor eyesight. Training for health care professionals is essential in ensuring that distress is minimised for these individuals and that care is made accessible. It is also essential that domiciliary and residential home care workers understand the profile of a person with autism and do not inadvertently cause stress by not recognising the person's needs.

> The staff in the care home where my mum is staying don't stick to time, come into her room without asking, don't tell her if builders are coming in to change the carpets or move furniture, and don't do what they've said they will. She hates it. (Adult daughter of older woman with autism)

> As a society the very young and the very old get more than their fair share of physical contact, because neurotypicals want to pat them. I saw some excellent carers [...] who, when they spoke to someone who was a bit vague, the hand would go down and they'd say, 'How are you today Mrs Brown?' 'All right, yes', and they'd be hand-holding her. That's absolutely right for a neurotypical; it's absolutely wrong for an autistic person [...] The horror of unwanted physical contact with people [...] you know they're doing this to be nice, but their fingers feel like ice on me. That's horrible, and so stressful. Some of

the most stressful and distressing things neurotypicals do is hug. (Lillian, National Autistic Society 2013a)

Physical and mental effects

Common features mentioned by older women were tiredness and fatigue. Although this is something generally associated with ageing, it appears that this perhaps comes on slightly earlier for women with autism – by the age of 40 – despite them being in otherwise good physical health. For some, getting through a whole day was too much without a nap. I am 100 per cent with them on this point and find the physical limitations that have come on quite quickly are both frustrating and a glorious liberation.

> I have needed a sleep in the afternoon since being around age 40. (Woman with autism)

> My health is good and I'm very fit for my age, but I get so tired and often have to fall asleep for a few hours in the daytime. (Woman with autism)

Along with a general physical tiredness, a number of women I have worked with have expressed a tiredness of holding it all together, of pretending to be someone else, of masking their autism. There is a real sense that the effort that these women have been making since childhood may have some long-term toll. They run out of steam; they simple can't do it anymore (or don't want to). The words used talk of fighting to 'survive'; these women have been battling to keep going in a world that feels alien and difficult. It seems that the combination of physical limitations associated with ageing and the number of years they have been 'fighting' can lead to a gradual slow-down once they reach their 40s and beyond.

> I was getting older and instead of things getting easier for me they were becoming more difficult as I had additional health issues to deal [with] (asthma, migraine disorder, hypothyroidism, IBS [Irritable Bowel Syndrome], neuropathy, etc.). This constant stress

was causing other health issues, including depression, and an overall lack of desire to live. I was just getting extremely tired of it all and tired of the fight to survive. My life was just one crisis after another. (Woman with autism)

I am tired of playing the role of someone who fits in, someone who can hold down a job and who wants what everyone else wants. I never wanted any of those things; I just did what I had to do to survive unnoticed and uncriticised. It has destroyed me mentally – and physically to some extent. I just want to retreat and live a small quiet life. I've had enough. (Woman with autism)

Lack of energy as I get older has limited the interests I pursue. This is disappointing, as there are many things that I have really enjoyed doing. Part of this, of course, is the depression that comes with Asperger's. Curtailing activities is par for the course. In an effort to get this energy back, I have started to exercise daily and work on my eating plan. (Woman with autism)

Being in crowds stresses me, like in a town, although it never used to. I don't know if the crowds have got bigger or if the older I've got my brain's processing of their movements has slowed down. I seem to find I use up so much energy trying to move among people. (Woman with autism)

I think I have gotten less interested in fitting in, less able to bite my tongue, less aware of gaffes, more tired, and far more resistant to change and unable to cope. (Woman with autism)

Other physical limitations mentioned mostly involved memory and a feeling of reduced brain-processing ability and speed.

One of the less positive things about my age is that the rate at which my brain processes information seems to have slowed down. I feel as if I have constant 'brain fog'. It seems to take [...] much longer for my brain's processing ability to kick in when I wake up. (National Autistic Society 2013a)

I can't remember facts at all, or names or people, places, TV programmes, characters in them or anything, and have got worse since reaching middle age. (Woman with autism)

Use [my] index finger to point at objects or directions to help brain know what to do. For instance, when at the grocery store I use my index finger to point at objects I'm trying to look for so I don't miss something I need to buy. When driving, I use my index finger to point at the direction I need to turn. (Woman with autism)

When I'm busy doing some activity, like getting ingredients together for a recipe, I can't respond to someone's question or conversation. I have to concentrate on doing what I'm doing to get it right. The same is also true when I'm typing an email to someone dear. I can't respond to someone's question or conversation. (Woman with autism)

A couple of women mentioned having increasing difficulties with speech.

I am finding it harder to speak coherently. Quite often I will say the wrong word or a made-up word, or I stutter. I have always been very strong linguistically and I find this upsetting and frightening as I don't know how it will progress. I am only in my 40s. [...] At times I say partial sentences, like that's all I can get out. My husband understands me, but I wonder if others would. When around other people, I usually just don't say anything unless I can speak with whole sentences. (Woman with autism)

Other physical changes mentioned included eyesight and hearing problems (which may be a natural consequence of ageing). These may have an additional impact for a person with autism who does not recognise faces well and has to look for other visual cues, or for someone who has always struggled to filter noise in busy environments. The loss of these faculties can greatly increase anxiety and make a person reluctant to leave the house and maintain an active life.

My eyesight causes me a lot of stress as I have so many pairs of glasses and forget them half the time [...] I mess about with a magnifying glass in the house to read labels on food as I can't locate my reading specs. (Woman with autism)

Hearing in large crowds is always difficult. It is hard to focus on what the one person is saying when you really hear all the other voices at the same time. Sometimes I find myself cupping my hand over the back of my ear to hear better. (Woman with autism)

Social impact

Seventy-three per cent of adults with autism over 55 years of age have three friends or fewer, with 65 per cent saying their main friends are their families or carers (National Autistic Society 2013b). It has been suggested that women with autism may have less interest in marriage and children (Ingudomnukul *et al.* 2007) and therefore we might conclude that more women with autism may age without families. We have also heard that women with autism have limited social networks and experience anxiety in social situations. These factors potentially lead to even greater isolation than is experienced by other older people. It is necessary to recognise that being older does not eliminate the features of autism, and socialising at any age will be difficult for these women, despite well-meaning invitations to day centres and lunch clubs.

Left to my own devices I will interact very little and not build relationships, but I am aware that I risk a very lonely old age if that continues. It's easy to get set in my ways and not seek others' company as I get older, but I do want to try and have some worthwhile relationships during the rest of my life. (Woman with autism)

The older I get the more lonely it feels as the people who really genuinely cared for me have gone [...] It's easier to stay home than make plans to go out, especially if it involves other people. We have our set activities and are comfortable in our own home. (Woman with autism)

The positive aspects of growing older

I got a real sense that the older women with autism had been able to come to terms with who they are. Due to their often very late diagnosis, self-acceptance had not been possible earlier in their lives. They talked about being able to assert what they needed to maintain their own well-being and feeling OK about that, rather than feeling bad about being perceived as different or difficult, which had been the case pre-diagnosis. After a lifetime of not being listened to, taken seriously or believed, some women were also able to obtain correct medication for their anxiety, depression and/or associated health conditions, which made life much easier. Having time to look after their health and well-being was also mentioned as being a positive result of becoming older.

> I am still very much a creature of habit and love routine. My ability to deal with change has improved a great deal as I have a better sense of perspective about what is the 'small stuff' that doesn't really matter. (Woman with autism)

> I find it's more important than ever to have my home as a place of sanctuary. I need to have things around me which make me feel calm and happy […] I think this is especially important the older you get. When the door buzzer goes, I ignore it when I want. The same goes for my telephone. If I don't feel like answering, I leave it. Email suits me just fine as it's not an intrusion into my peace and I can reply when I feel like it. (National Autistic Society 2013a)

> My health has improved as I've got older, partly due to correct medication and more recently due to taking up a fairly intensive gym regime. I'm fitter than I've ever been and hope to maintain that as the years go by. (Woman with autism)

> I'm finding that being an older woman in today's society renders me somewhat invisible, especially as I don't conform to my gender stereotype by wearing overtly feminine clothes and make-up, and I find this invisibility a relief and advantageous in that I have less unwelcome, intrusive attention to deal with. (Woman with autism)

For some older women with autism there is a sense of feeling comfortable with themselves for the first time (Simone 2010) and feeling more able to be their 'real' selves, almost becoming 'more autistic' in the process. Several women mentioned that they felt this way and that this had been surprising both to their families and the professionals around them. They felt that others had expected them to become more 'normal' and that this had not happened (Simone 2010). This was combined with the physical and mental decline in function mentioned above: 'I can't do it anymore; I don't want to do it anymore'. Eccentricities became more pronounced and tolerances were reduced. Some mentioned feeling younger than their age and, perhaps due to a lesser need to conform to social norms, were able to engage in activities and with people not traditionally associated with older women. Women with autism often don't see any reason why they shouldn't do something due to age, gender or any other factor. This is enormously liberating and the reason why you'll find older women with autism doing all sorts of crazy stuff!

> I now go to roller discos and find it has really cheered me up as most of the people there are a bit younger than me. There are some people older too though, so I'm not like the odd one out or anything. It's good to keep joining things that are not just for older people. (Woman with autism)

> I still feel and act much younger than my age. If I am talking to women in their 20s I feel I can laugh at silly things, and if I can have a bit of a lark playing a game of ten-pin bowling with a group of 25-year-old Aspie girls then I feel so much better afterwards. (National Autistic Society 2013a)

> God, what a relief being older is. I've become invisible. No-one expects anything of me anymore – I'm just old. Sad though that is in some ways, it's also a huge liberation: I can do whatever I like and nobody cares. (Woman with autism)

> There are problems I haven't been able to rectify, but I know how to be kind to myself. When I get home, electric lights go off and I light candles. I burn oils because they calm me. I am learning how to

slow down the chatter that runs through my head and I am looking for the key to a full night of sleep. I might never be at ease with you, but I am more at ease with myself. (National Autistic Society 2013a)

For those who had raised children, older years can feel like a huge relief of stress and responsibility as those children have grown up and daily care for them is no longer required.

Grandma has autism

Being a grandparent with autism is a completely unresearched area. There may be expectations that women will fulfil a grandparent's role following decades of caring for their own children, when in fact they may be exhausted and wanting to spend time focusing on themselves. The assumption and expectation of women as willing and natural nurturers can rear its head again when considering the role of grandmother and lead to further disappointment when Grandma is off and away kite-surfing (or long-distance cycling, kick-boxing and paint-balling, in my case). I have twin grandsons who are a great source of joy in my life, but the old adage of being able to give them back is so true. I feel that I can be a good Grandma because my obligations to them are short, time-bound and usually planned in advance. The round-the-clock job description of parenting was not my forte, but I can do 'temping' parenting as a grandmother. I have patience, tolerance and energy purely because I know that my duties are finite.

> When my youngest child reached 18, I felt a very palpable sense of a weight being lifted. I know they still need me, but not every minute of every day. I have started to look forward now to a life for me without them. I'm glad I had them, but it was desperately hard and no one knew. (Woman with autism)

> I am a much better granny than I was a mother. I can enjoy the good bits but I don't have to worry about getting everything right for them – that is someone else's job. It allows me to be so much more relaxed than I was with my own kids. (Woman with autism)

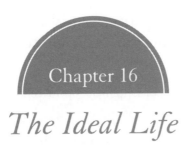

Chapter 16

The Ideal Life

What I crave most of all is time [...] to indulge my special interests and acquire new ones. I'd like to be able to [...] pursu[e] things that make me happy and, if possible, also mak[e] the world a kinder, more tolerant and compassionate place for animals and vulnerable people.

WOMAN WITH AUTISM

To sum up all the thoughts, life experiences and knowledge that the women with autism I questioned have gathered, I wanted to ask them where this has led them. Now they knew who they were and why they'd had the lives they'd had, what conclusions had they drawn about what made them feel well, happy and fulfilled? If obligation, social conformity and money were no object, what would they do? These are a only a few responses from a community of millions of individuals with their own dreams and carefully made plans, so, like anything in this book, should not be taken as a definitive statement of fact about women and girls with autism, but may give a flavour of what matters to these people.

WHAT WOULD IMPROVE THE QUALITY OF YOUR LIFE?

Better social skills and understanding of people. I'm nearly 50 and still find it a minefield. (Woman with autism)

Help with keeping my flat tidy or help with being more organised. (Woman with autism)

Greater provision around the country of some sort of support groups for older AS [Asperger Syndrome] people would help. (Woman with autism)

Possibly some sort of helpline/drop-in centre. Advice on getting jobs etc. (Woman with autism)

I think there needs to be support with romantic relationships, especially for younger women. Someone they can ask questions and not feel embarrassed. (Woman with autism)

WHAT WOULD YOUR 'IDEAL LIFE' LOOK LIKE?

Plenty of pets, especially dogs. Work from home with some interaction with others. Own house and garden. (Woman with autism)

My ideal life would be where I had a partner and someone to spend my leisure time with, or some of it. I would have a job that didn't stress me and a few good friends. (Woman with autism)

I would travel, a lot. I love to travel, all by myself. (Woman with autism)

I would like to be financially secure so as not to have to worry about how I will earn a living in the future. I would like enough money to be able to live comfortably rather than in luxury. (Woman with autism)

Three homes (although I guess that is pretty luxurious!). One in rural England – small, old, stone cottage on the outskirts of a village or small town near the coast; another in central London – a one-bed flat so that I could visit the theatre and museums more often and not have to worry about travelling home on the tube/train; and a third somewhere warm, probably Spain or Lanzarote – again a small, traditional, stone-built property within a village community where I could spend December to March. (Woman with autism)

I need to live alone but would like to live within walking distance of my sister or a close friend for support [...] If I could live independently among a community of like-minded individuals who share my special interests that would be brilliant. (Woman with autism)

I consider any time spent in research and gaining a greater understanding of myself, exploring my creative side in practical projects and just messing about outdoors in nature to be time well spent. (Woman with autism)

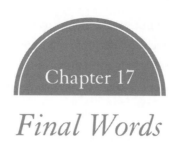

Chapter 17

Final Words

I know I am valuable and have a place in the world. I have become my own person and truly like who I am. The process has been a difficult one and I know that my being egocentric is just too much for some people. How much more comfortable humans are with those of us who conform to expectation, who fit in with conventional 'norms' and who are not an embarrassment.

LAWSON (1998, P.117)

Women with autism are a resilient bunch: often anxious, depressed, overwhelmed, but continuing to work at making sense of a world that makes no sense; trying to fit into a world where they just don't fit. You cannot imagine what that feels like every minute of every day, but you need to try.

Young women with autism need to be taught, encouraged and pushed (gently) to achieve whatever they want. Autism is not an excuse for limiting aspirations – older, very late-diagnosed women with autism prove that. They don't need wrapping in cotton wool. They need to understand their anxieties and the world they live in, and be taught how to make the best of it.

These women need opportunities to speak to each other and find their own tribe, their own community. This is a place where they can share their trials and tribulations and not get the response, 'You did what?', but instead hear, 'Yeah, I do that too'. This can make all the difference between self-esteem and self-hatred.

The first step is for professionals to understand that the profile shows itself differently in females than in males. You have to work a bit harder to find it, but it's there. And just because it's not too visible, doesn't mean it's not 'severe'.

Increased access to diagnosis is the first step to enable women to get the validation and access to services that they need.

Clinicians: You are the gatekeepers to a much greater quality of life for these girls and women. Learn what to ask, listen to them, look for the autism beneath the facade.

Education professionals, support workers and families: It may be more than just 'teenage girl stuff', 'a neurotic' (that was how I was described) or 'shyness'. It may be something else. Just because she's quiet and not causing you any trouble, don't overlook her. She's not like other girls; don't judge her unfavourably against yourself (as a woman) or other girls/women. She thinks differently; keep an open mind.

Girls and women with autism: You're fine exactly as you are. Yes, you're a bit weird, but that's perfectly alright. You might not feel much like a 'woman', but that's OK too – most of us don't. And you're totally right about handbags. You only need one, and that's a rucksack. And don't ever, EVER compare yourself to a neurotypical (NT) girl or woman. They are a different species and you'll only feel inadequate and bad about yourself. Find your tribe – online, in groups at comic conventions. Find people who are delighted that you are you. And you should be delighted that you are you too because when you're 70, you'll still be skateboarding, you'll look amazing (from all those years of not ruining your skin with make-up) and you'll realise that all those things you worried about don't matter at all.

For my final words, let's leave it to the women without whom this book would have been pretty dull. I asked the older women for their words of wisdom to their younger 'sisters' making their way through the world. After all, they had been there and got the T-shirt, often without any diagnosis or support. Their words were strong, uplifting and encouraged persistence, self-knowledge and getting out there and finding a life.

Keep facing up to your fears and get new experiences. I always loved the book *Feel the Fear and Do it Anyway* by Susan Jeffers. (Woman with autism)

Autism is just a thing that you have, it doesn't have to define you. It's not the most interesting thing about you. Know your limits and explore as much as you can within them. AS [Asperger Syndrome] doesn't have to be a prison! (Woman with autism)

It's okay, don't sweat it. Just be pro-active to do what you can and go with the rest of the flow. Heh, read this book! (Woman with autism)

Be yourself. You're awesome just as you are. (Woman with autism)

References

American Psychiatric Association (2013) *Diagnostic and Statistical Manual of Mental Disorders, Fifth Edition, DSM-5*. Arlington, VA: American Psychiatric Association.

Attwood, T. (2007) *Complete Guide to Asperger's Syndrome*. London: Jessica Kingsley Publishers.

Attwood, T. (2012) 'Girls with Asperger's Syndrome: early diagnosis is critical'. *Autism Asperger's Digest* July/August 2012. Available at www.autismdigest.com/girls-with-a. Accessed on 22 November 2014.

Attwood, T. (2013) 'Girls' Questionnaire for Autism Spectrum Conditions (GQ-ASC)'. Unpublished. For more details, contact Professor Attwood via his website www.tonyattwood.com.au.

Attwood, T., Bolick, T., Faherty, C., Iland. L. *et al.* (2006) *Asperger's and Girls*. Arlington, TX: Future Horizons, Inc.

Autism and Developmental Disabilities Monitoring Network (2014) 'Prevalence of autism spectrum disorder among children aged 8 years – Autism and Developmental Disabilities Monitoring Network, 11 sites, United States, 2010'. *Morbidity and Mortality Weekly Report Surveillance Summaries 63*, 02, 1–21.

Autism Women Matter (2013) *Autism Women Matter Survey, 2013*. Autism Women Matter. Available at www.autismwomenmatter.org.uk/survey. Accessed on 22 November 2014.

Baron-Cohen, S. (2002) 'The extreme male brain theory of autism'. *Trends in Cognitive Science 6*, 6, 248–54.

Baron-Cohen, S., Jaffa, T., Davies, S., Auyeung, B., Allison, C. and Wheelwright, S. (2013) 'Do girls with anorexia nervosa have elevated autistic traits?' *Molecular Autism 4*, 1, 24.

Bejerot, S., Eriksson, J.M., Bonde, S., Carlstrom, K., Humble, M.B. and Eriksson, E. (2012) 'The extreme male brain revisited: gender coherence in adults with autism spectrum disorder'. *British Journal of Psychiatry 201*, 2, 116–23.

Bölte, S., Duketis, E., Poustka, F. and Holtmann, M. (2011) 'Sex differences in cognitive domains and their clinical correlates in higher-functioning autism spectrum disorders'. *Autism 15*, 4, 497–511.

Carter, A.S., Black, D.O., Tewani, S., Connolly, C.E., Kadlec, M.B. and Tager-Flusberg, H. (2007) 'Sex differences in toddlers with autism spectrum disorders'. *Journal of Autism and Developmental Disorders 37*, 1, 86–97.

Cassidy, S., Bradley, P., Robinson, J., Allison, C., McHugh, M. and Baron-Cohen, S. (2014) 'Suicidal ideation and suicide plans or attempts in adults with Asperger's syndrome attending a specialist diagnostic clinic: a clinical cohort study'. *The Lancet Psychiatry 1*, 2, 142–7.

Craig, M.C., Zaman, S.H., Daly, E.M., Cutter, W.J. *et al.* (2007) 'Women with autistic-spectrum disorder: magnetic resonance imaging study of brain anatomy'. *British Journal of Psychiatry 191*, 224–8.

de Vries, A. L., Noens, I.L., Cohen-Kettenis, P. T., van Berckelaer-Onnes, I.A. and Doreleijers, T.A. (2010) 'Autism Spectrum Disorders in gender dysphoric children and adolescents'. *Journal of Autism and Developmental Disorders*, August 2010; 40, 8, 930–936.

Eaton, L. (2012) 'Under the radar and behind the scenes: the perspectives of mothers with daughters on the autism spectrum'. *Good Autism Practice 13*, 2, 9–17.

Fombonne, E. (2005) 'The changing epidemiology of autism'. *Journal of Applied Research in Intellectual Disabilities 18*, 4, 281–94.

Frazier T.W. *et al.* (2014) 'Behavioral and cognitive characteristics of females and males with autism in the Simons Simplex Collection'. *Journal of the American Academy of Child and Adolescent Psychiatry 53*, 329–340.

Gaus, V. (2007) *Cognitive Behavioural Therapy for Adult Asperger Syndrome*. New York, NY: The Guilford Press.

Gaus, V. (2011) *Living Well on the Spectrum*. New York, NY: The Guilford Press.

Giarelli, E., Wiggins, L.D., Rice, C.E., Levy, S.E. *et al.* (2010) 'Sex differences in the evaluation and diagnosis of autism spectrum disorders among children'. *Disability and Health Journal 3*, 2, 107–16.

Gilmour, L., Melike Schalomon, P. and Smith, V. (2012) 'Sexuality in a community based sample of adults with autism spectrum disorder'. *Research in Autism Spectrum Disorders 6*, 1, 313–18.

Gould, J. (2014). Personal communication. 10 January 2014.

Gould, J. and Ashton-Smith, J. (2011) 'Missed diagnosis or misdiagnosis? Girls and women on the autism spectrum'. *Good Autism Practice 12*, 1, 34–41.

Hartley, S.L. and Sikora, D.M. (2009) 'Sex differences in autism spectrum disorder: an examination of developmental functioning, autistic symptoms, and coexisting behaviour problems in toddlers'. *Journal of Autism and Developmental Disorders* 39, 12, 1715–22.

Head, A.M., McGillivray, J.A. and Stokes, M.A. (2014) 'Gender differences in emotionality and sociability in children with autism spectrum disorders'. *Molecular Autism 5*, 19.

Hendrickx, S. and Newton, K. (2007) *Asperger Syndrome – A Love Story*. London: Jessica Kingsley Publishers.

Hendrickx, S. (2008) *Love, Sex and Long-term Relationships: What People with Asperger Syndrome Really Really Want*. London: Jessica Kingsley Publishers.

Hendrickx, S. (2009) *Asperger Syndrome and Employment: What People with Asperger Syndrome Really Really Want*. London: Jessica Kingsley Publishers.

Holliday Willey, L. (2001) *Asperger Syndrome in the Family*. London: Jessica Kingsley Publishers.

Holliday Willey, L. (2012) *Safety Skills for Asperger Women: How to Save a Perfectly Good Female Life*. London: Jessica Kingsley Publishers.

Holliday Willey, L. (2014) *Pretending to be Normal: Living with Asperger's Syndrome*. London: Jessica Kingsley Publishers.

Hurley, E. (ed.) (2014) *Ultraviolet Voices: Stories of Women on the Autism Spectrum*. Birmingham: Autism West Midlands.

Impact Initiatives, Asperger's Voice Self-Advocacy Group & West Sussex Asperger Awareness Group (2013) *Mental Health Services for Adults with Asperger's Syndrome and HFA in West Sussex: A Quality Check*. Littlehampton: Impact Initiatives.

Ingudomnukul, E., Baron-Cohen, S., Wheelwright, S. and Knickmeyer, R. (2007) 'Elevated rates of testosterone-related disorders in women with autism spectrum conditions'. *Hormones and Behavior 51*, 5, 597–604.

Jacquemont, S., Coe, B.P., Hersch, M., Duyzend, M.H., *et al.* (2014) 'A higher mutational burden in females supports a "female protective model" in neurodevelopmental disorders'. *American Journal of Human Genetics 94*, 3, 415–25.

Jansen, H. and Rombout, B. (2014) *Autipower: Successful Living and Working with an Autism Spectrum Disorder*. London: Jessica Kingsley Publishers.

Joss, L. (2013) 'Is Anorexia the Female Asperger's?' Available at www. autismdailynewscast.com/is-anorexia-the-female-aspergers/5518/laurel-joss. Accessed on 22 November 2014.

Kanner, L. (1943) 'Autistic disturbances of affective contact'. *Nervous Child 2*, 217–50.

Kearns Miller, J. (2003) *Women from Another Planet?* Bloomington, IN: 1st Books Library.

Knickmeyer, R.C., Wheelwright, S. and Baron-Cohen, S. (2008) 'Sex-typical play: masculinization/defeminization in girls with an autism spectrum condition'. *Journal of Autism and Developmental Disorders 38*, 6, 1028–35.

Kopp, S. and Gillberg, C. (1992) 'Girls with social deficits and learning problems: autism, atypical Asperger syndrome or a variant of these conditions'. *European Child and Adolescent Psychiatry 1*, 2, 89–99.

Kopp, S. and Gillberg, C. (2011) 'The Autism Spectrum Screening Questionnaire (ASSQ)-Revised Extended Version (ASSQ-REV): an instrument for better capturing the autism phenotype in girls? A preliminary study involving 191 clinical cases and community controls'. *Journal Research in Developmental Disabilities 32*, 6, 2875–88.

Kreiser, N.L. and White, S.W. (2014) 'ASD in females: are we overstating the gender difference in diagnosis?' *Clinical Child and Family Psychology Review 17*, 1, 67–84.

Lai, M.C., Lombardo, M.V., Pasco, G., Ruigrok, A.N. *et al.* (2011) 'A behavioral comparison of male and female adults with high functioning autism spectrum conditions'. *PLOS One 6*, 6, e20835.

Lai, M.C., Lombardo, M.V., Suckling, J., Ruigrok, A.N. *et al.* (2013) 'Biological sex affects the neurobiology of autism'. *Brain 136*, 9, 2799–815.

Lawson, W. (1998) *Life Behind Glass: A Personal Account of Autism Spectrum Disorder.* London: Jessica Kingsley Publishers.

Lawson, W. (2014). Personal communication 9 October 2014.

Lemon, J.M., Gargaro, B., Enticott, P.G. and Rinehart, N.J. (2011) 'Executive functioning in autism spectrum disorders: a gender comparison of response inhibition'. *Journal of Autism and Developmental Disorders 41*, 3, 352–6.

Lord, C., Schopler, E. and Revicki, D. (1982) 'Sex differences in autism'. *Journal of Autism and Developmental Disorders 12*, 4, 317–30.

Mandy, W. (2013) *DSM-5 May Better Serve Girls with Autism.* New York: Simons Foundation Autism Research Initiative. Available at www.sfari.org/news-and-opinion/specials/2013/dsm-5-special-report/dsm-5-may-better-serve-girls-with-autism. Accessed on 22 November 2014.

Mandy, W., Chilvers, R., Chowdhury, U., Salter, G., Seigal, A. and Skuse, D. (2012) 'Sex differences in autism spectrum disorder: evidence from a large sample of children and adolescents'. *Journal of Autism and Developmental Disorders 42*, 7, 1304–13.

Marshall, T. *Aspienwomen: Adult Women with Asperger Syndrome. Moving towards a female profile of Asperger Syndrome.* Available at http://taniaannmarshall.wordpress.com/2013/03/26/moving-towards-a-female-profile-the-unique-characteristics-abilities-and-talents-of-asperwomen-adult-women-with-asperger-syndrome/, accessed on 6 November 2014.

McCarthy, M.M., Arnold, A.P., Ball, G.F., Blaustein, J.D. and De Vries, G.J. (2012) 'Sex differences in the brain: the not so inconvenient truth'. *Journal of Neuroscience 32*, 7, 2241–7.

McLennan, J.D., Lord, C. and Schopler, E. (1993) 'Sex differences in higher functioning people with autism'. *Journal of Autism and Developmental Disorders 23*, 2, 217–27.

National Autistic Society (2013a) 'Autism and Ageing: Older People's Stories'. Available at www.autism.org.uk/living-with-autism/adults-with-autism-or-asperger-syndrome/autism-and-ageing/older-peoples-stories.aspx. Accessed on 22 November 2014.

National Autistic Society (2013b) *Getting On: Growing Older with Autism: A Policy Report*. London: National Autistic Society.

National Collaborating Centre for Mental Health (2012) *Autism: The NICE Guideline on Recognition, Referral, Diagnosis and Management of Adults on the Autism Spectrum*. London: The British Psychological Society and The Royal College of Psychiatrists.

Nichols, S., Moravcik, G.M. and Tetenbaum, S.P. (2009) *Girls Growing up on the Autism Spectrum*. London: Jessica Kingsley Publishers.

Nyden, A., Hjelmquist, E. and Gilberg, C. (2000) 'Autism spectrum and attention deficit disorders in girls: some neuropsychological aspects'. *European Child and Adolescent Psychiatry 9*, 3, 180–5.

Oldershaw, A., Treasure, J., Hambrook, D., Tchanturia, K. and Schmidt, U. (2011) 'Is anorexia nervosa a version of autism spectrum disorders?' *European Eating Disorders Review 19*, 6, 462–74.

Pelz-Sherman, D. (2014) 'Supporting breastfeeding among women on the autistic spectrum'. *Clinical Lactation, 5*, 2, 62–6.

Pohl, A., Cassidy, S., Auyeung, B. and Baron-Cohen, S. (2014) 'Uncovering steroidopathy in women with autism: a latent class analysis'. *Molecular Autism 5*, 27.

Riley-Hall, E. (2012) *Parenting Girls on the Autism Spectrum*. London: Jessica Kingsley Publishers.

Ruigrok, A.N.V., Salimi-Khorshidi, G., Lai, M-C., Baron-Cohen, S. *et al.* (2014) 'A meta-analysis of sex differences in human brain structure'. *Neuroscience & Biobehavioral Reviews 39*, 34–50.

Russell, G., Steer, C. and Golding, J. (2011) 'Social and demographic factors that influence the diagnosis of autistic spectrum disorders'. *Social Psychiatry and Psychiatric Epidemiology 46*, 12, 1283–93.

Simone, R. (2010) *Aspergirls*. London: Jessica Kingsley Publishers.

Stewart, C. (2012) '"Where can we be what we are?": the experiences of girls with Asperger syndrome and their mothers'. *Good Autism Practice, 13*, 1, 40–8.

Tinsley, M. and Hendrickx, S. (2008) *Asperger Syndrome and Alcohol: Drinking to Cope.* London: Jessica Kingsley Publishers.

Tsai, L.Y. and Beisler, J.M. (1983) 'The development of sex differences in infantile autism'. *British Journal of Psychiatry 142*, 373–8.

University of Cambridge (2013) *Autism Affects Different Parts of the Brain in Women and Men.* Cambridge: University of Cambridge. Available at www.cam.ac.uk/research/news/autism-affects-different-parts-of-the-brain-in-women-and-men. Accessed on 22 November 2014.

van Wijngaarden-Cremers, P.J.M. (2012) 'Gender differences and its impact on women with ASD'. Women and Girls on the Autism Spectrum Conference 2012, National Autistic Society.

Volkmar, F.R., Szatmari, P. and Sparrow, S.S. (1993) 'Sex differences in pervasive developmental disorders'. *Journal of Autism and Developmental Disorders 23*, 4, 579–91.

Wagner, S. (2006) 'Educating the Female Student with Asperger's.' In Attwood, T., Bolick, T., Faherty, C., Iland. L. *et al. Asperger's and Girls.* Arlington, TX: Future Horizons, Inc.

Wing, L. (1981) 'Sex ratios in early childhood autism and related conditions'. *Psychiatry Research 5*, 2, 129–37.

Wylie, P. (2014) *Very Late Diagnosis of Asperger Syndrome.* London: Jessica Kingsley Publishers.

Zahn-Waxler, C., Shirtcliff, E.A. and Marceau, K. (2008) 'Disorders of childhood and adolescence: gender and psychopathology'. *Annual Review of Clinical Psychology 4*, 275–303.

Index